Keto Chaffle Cookbook

An Easy Guide to Make Delicious Chaffles with Low Carb
Recipes to Lose Weight, Improve Your Health and Satisfy your
soul. With Pictures!

By

Camila Rivera

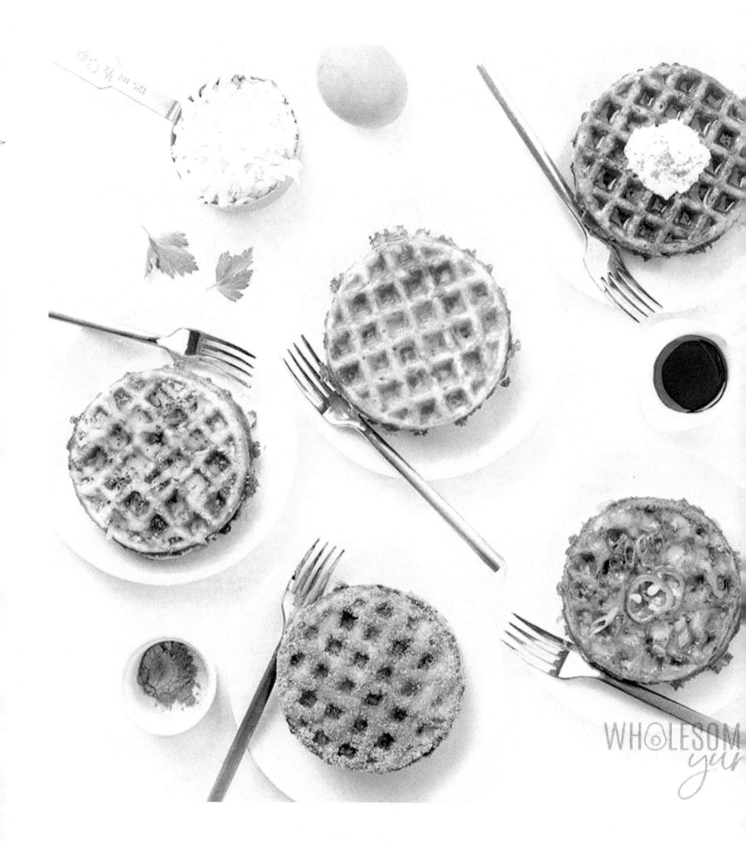

TABLE OF CONTENTS

Introduction

Ketogenic refers to a low-carbohydrate diet. The aim is to eat more calories from f
and protein while eating fewer calories from carbohydrates. The carbohydrates tha
are easiest to digest, such as starch, pastries, soda, and white bread, are the first
to go. When you consume fewer than 50 g of carbohydrates a day, your body easi
runs out of energy. This normally takes three or four days. Then you'll begin to
break down fat and protein for energy, potentially resulting in weight loss. Ketosis
the term for this state. It's crucial to remember that the ketogenic diet is a short-
term diet designed to help you lose weight rather than change your lifestyle. A
ketogenic diet is more often used to reduce weight, although it may also be used t
treat medical problems such as epilepsy. It can even benefit those suffering from
heart failure, some brain disorders, and even acne, although further study is
required. Since the keto diet contains too much fat, adherents must ingest fat at
every meal time. In a normal 2K-calorie diet, that would seem like 165 g of fat, 40
g of carbohydrates, and 75 g of protein. The exact ratio, on the other hand, is
determined by your basic requirements. Nuts (walnuts, almonds), avocados, seeds
olive oil and tofu are among the healthier unsaturated fats allowed on the keto die
However, oils (coconut, palm), butter, lard, and peanut butter all contain high
amounts of saturated fats. Protein is an essential aspect of the keto diet, although
is also difficult to discern between protein items that are lean and protein products
rich in fat(saturated), such as beef, bacon, and pork. What for fruits and
vegetables? While fruits are generally rich in carbohydrates, unique fruits may be
obtained in limited quantities (generally berries) Leafy greens (like kale, chard,
Swiss chard, and spinach), broccoli, cauliflower, asparagus, tomatoes, brussels
sprouts, bell peppers, garlic, cucumbers, mushrooms, summer squashes, as well a
celery are also rich in carbohydrates. One cup of sliced broccoli includes about six
carbohydrates. At the same time, there are several possible keto hazards, such as
liver deficiency, liver complications, constipation, kidney disorders, and so on. As a
result, we can also keep our Keto diet portions in check.

Understanding The Ketogenic Diet

This chapter delves into the Ketogenic diet in depth. The chapter further discusses which foods to consume on the Keto diet and which foods to stop while on this diet. The Keto diet is often explained in-depth, including how it functions and what health advantages it provides.

The ketogenic diet (or keto diet) is a high-fat, low-carbohydrate diet with various health benefits. Evidently, more than 20 studies suggest that this form of diet will help you lose weight and boost your wellbeing. Diabetes patients, epilepsy patients, patients suffering from Alzheimer's disease, as well as cancer can all benefit from ketogenic diets.

1.1 What is Keto?

The ketogenic diet is a very low carbohydrate, high-fat diet that has a lot in common with the Atkins diet and other low-carb diets. It necessitates a significant reduction of carbohydrate consumption and a replacement with fat. This reduction of carbohydrates puts the body into a metabolic condition known as ketosis. As this occurs, the body's energy production of fat-burning skyrockets. In addition, it converts fat into ketones in the liver, which will supply energy to the brain. Ketogenic diets can result in substantial reductions in insulin as well as blood sugar levels. This, along with the increased ketones, has numerous health benefits.

Ketogenic Diets Come in Many Forms

There are a few variations of the ketogenic diet, including:

The traditional ketogenic diet consists of a diet that is low in carbs, mild in protein, and strong in fats. It usually has a 75 percent fat content, a 5% carbohydrate content, and a 20% protein content.

The cyclic ketogenic diet entails high-carb reefed cycles, such as five ketogenic days accompanied by two days of high carbohydrate use.

A ketogenic diet with particular goals: The diet requires carbs to be inserted between exercises.

Protein-rich ketogenic diet: This is comparable to a normal keto diet, but it contai extra protein. Usually, the ratio is 60 percent fat, 5% sugars, and 35 percent prote

However, only normal and protein-rich ketogenic diets have been extensively studie More complex keto diets, such as targeted or cyclic keto, are mainly utilized bodybuilders and athletes.

Ketogenic Diet Health Benefits

In fact, the keto diet first gained popularity as a means of treating neurologi conditions, such as epilepsy. Following that, research has shown that diet can he with a broad variety of health issues:

Heart disease: The keto diet has been found to decrease risk factors such as bo fat, blood sugar, HDL cholesterol and blood pressure.

Alzheimer's disease: The ketogenic diet can ease Alzheimer's symptoms while s delaying the disease's progression.

Epilepsy: Research has demonstrated that a ketogenic diet can significantly redu seizures in children with epileptic seizures.

Cancer: The diet is actually being used to control a number of diseases and to del tumor development.

Acne: Lower insulin levels, as well as less sugar or fried food diets, will aid ac recovery.

Parkinson's disease: According to one report, diet can help relieve the effects Parkinson's disease.

Brain injuries: One study found that the diet would also increase concussions a improve recovery after a brain injury.

Polycystic ovary syndrome: A ketogenic diet may help lower insulin levels and can helpful in the treatment of polycystic ovary syndrome.

What foods can you consume on a ketogenic diet?

The majority of your meals will revolve around the following foods:

- Salmon, mackerel and tuna are representations of fatty fish.
- Look for pastured eggs, whole eggs, or omega-3 eggs.
- Seek for grass-fed butter plus cream wherever possible.
- Red meat, ham, sausage, turkey, bacon, chicken and steak are all examples of meat.
- Non-processed cheese (goat, cheddar, mozzarella, blue, or cream).
- Flax seeds, walnuts, almonds, pumpkin seeds, chia seeds and other nuts and beans
- Avocado oil, olive oil and coconut oil are the other safe oils.
- Salt, spices and pepper, as well as a variety of herbs, may be used as condiments.
- Avocados: entire avocados or guacamole made freshly.
- Low-carb vegetables including greens, tomatoes, onions, peppers and other related veggies.

Foods to avoid on a ketogenic diet include:

Carbohydrate-rich diets can be avoided as much as possible.

The following is a selection of items that must be eliminated or reduced on a ketogenic diet:

- Sugary drink, ice cream, soda, smoothies, cake, candy and other sugary items
- Wheat, pasta, cereals, rice, and other wheat-based products are examples of starches or grains.
- Sweet potatoes, parsnips, parsnips, potatoes, carrots and other tubers & root vegetables
- Reduced-calorie or low-fat foods are extremely processed and abundant in carbohydrates.
- Fruit: All fruits, with the exception of tiny bits of berries like strawberries.
- Chickpeas, lentils, peas, kidney beans, and other legumes or beans
- Some sauces/condiments: They are also high in unhealthy fat and sugar.
- Unhealthy fats: Limit the intake to mayonnaise, processed vegetable oils, and other processed fats.

- Alcohol: Because of their carb content, certain alcoholic beverages will sha[...] you out of ketosis.
- Dietary ingredients that are sugar-free: Alcohols, which are often rich in suga[...] may influence ketone levels in certain situations. These objects seem to ha[...] passed through a lot of refining as well.

1.2 What is the Keto diet, and how does it work?

The "ketogenic" keto diet consists of consuming a moderate level of protein, a hea[...] amount of fat, and relatively little carbohydrates; also, the fruit is forbidden. As f[...] every diet fad, the advantages to adherents include improved vitality, weig[...] reduction, and mental clarity. Is the ketogenic diet, though, what it's cracked up [...] be?

Dietitians and nutritionists are quiet on the topic. Low-carb diets like keto appear [...] assist with weight loss in the short term, but they are no more successful than a[...] other self-help or conventional diet. They still don't seem to be enhancing athle[...] results.

The ketogenic diet was created to treat epilepsy instead of losing weight. In t[...] 1920s, physicians found that holding people on low-carb diets induced their bodies [...] use fat as the predominant fuel source rather than glucose. When only fat is availab[...] for the body to combust or burn, the body converts fats to fatty acids, which are th[...] converted to ketones, which can be used and taken up to power the body's cells.

Currently, feeding the body exclusively ketones prevents epilepsy for unclear cause[...] However, with the advent of anti-seizure medicines, few patients with epilepsy re[...] on ketogenic diets anymore, while certain people who may not respond to medicatio[...] may benefit. Low carb diets like the Atkins diet, which gained popularity in the ea[...] 2000s, also spawned keto diets for weight loss. In comparison, all groups of meatie[...] meal diets restrict carbohydrates. This diet does not have a set structure, althoug[...] most routines provide for fewer than fifty grams of carbs per day.

A keto diet causes the body to enter a state known as ketosis, in which the body[...] cells become completely reliant on ketones for nutrition. It's not exactly clear th[...]

this leads to weight loss, but ketosis decreases appetite and can affect hunger-controlling hormones, including insulin. As a consequence, proteins and fats can keep humans fuller longer than sugars, resulting in lower net calorie intake.

In one head-to-head comparison, researchers looked at 48 separate diet trials in which subjects were randomly allocated to one of the well-known diets. Low-carb diets like South Beach, Atkins, and Zone, as well as low-fat diets like Ornish diets and portion restriction diets like Weight Watchers and Jenny Craig, were among the options.

Every diet resulted in greater weight loss than almost no diet after six months, according to the results. Low-carb and low-fat dieters lost almost equal amounts of weight as compared to non-dieters, with low-carb dieters losing 19 pounds on average versus low-fat dieters dropping 17.6 pounds (7.99 kilograms). At 12 months, both diet styles displayed symptoms of dropping off, with low-fat and low-carb dieters being 16 pounds (7.27 kg) smaller on average than non-dieters.

There were few differences in weight reduction within the diets of designated people. This is in line with the practice of recommending every diet that an individual practice in order to lose weight.

Another study of well-known diets discovered the Atkins diet, which results in greater weight loss than merely teaching people about portion control. Nevertheless, several of the scientific researched about this low-carb diet featured licensed dietitians assisting respondents in making food decisions, rather than the self-directed approach used by most people. This has been seen in other diet studies, according to the researchers, and the tests' results seem to be more positive in the real world than the weight loss.

Finally, a simple comparison between low-carb versus low-fat dieting revealed that there was a statistically significant difference in the amount of weight lost over a year. Low-carbohydrate dieters dropped an average of 13 pounds (6 kg), compared to 11.7 pounds for low-fat dieters (5.3 kg).

Ketogenic diets may help us lose weight, but they are no more successful than other diet methods. Since carbohydrate reserves in the body comprise water molecules, the bulk of the weight lost during the early stages of a ketogenic diet is water weight.

This gives the scale an exciting amount at first, but weight reduction slows down w
time.

What are the keto effects, and how can they help?

The advantages of a keto diet are close to that of other high-fat, low-carb diets, b
it tends to be more successful than centrist low-carb diets. Keto is a low-carb, hig
fat diet that maximizes health benefits. However, it will slightly raise the likelihood
complications.

Aid in weight loss

Weight reduction can be improved by converting the body into a fat-burning devic
Insulin levels – the hormone that retains fat – are falling rapidly, suggesting that
burning has risen dramatically. This seems to make it much easier to lose bodyweig
without going hungry.

More than thirty high-quality observational studies show that low-carb and keto die
are more effective than other diets at losing weight.

Reverse type 2 diabetes by regulating blood sugar

A ketogenic diet has been shown in research to be successful in the treatment of ty
2 diabetes, with total disease reversal occurring in certain instances. It makes perfe
sense since keto removes the need for therapy, lowers blood sugar levels, a
eliminates the potential negative consequences of high insulin levels.

Since a keto diet will reverse type 2 diabetes, it is likely to be helpful in preventi
and reversing pre-diabetes. Keep in mind that "reversal" in this context refers
changing the disease, improving glucose tolerance, and reducing the need for ca
It may be so drastically altered that after therapy, blood pressure returns to norm
with time. In this context, reversal refers to progressing or deteriorating in t
reverse direction of the condition. Changes in your lifestyle, on the other side, ju
succeed if you bring them into effect. If a person returns to the way of life he or s
has before diabetes type 2 appeared and advanced, it is possible that success wou
return with time.

Improve your mental and physical performance:

Some people use ketogenic diets to boost their mental performance. It's also normal for people to feel more energized while they're in ketosis.

They don't need nutritional carbs for the brain on keto. It runs on ketones 24 hours a day, seven days a week, with a small amount of glucose synthesized in the liver. Carbohydrates are not necessary for the diet. As a result, ketosis leads to a steady flow of food (ketones) to the brain, avoiding significant blood sugar spikes. This will also assist with improved focus and attention, as well as clearing brain fog and improving mental awareness.

Epilepsy Treatment

The keto diet has been used to manage epilepsy since the 19th and 20th centuries and has proved to be effective. It has historically been used mainly for adolescents, although in recent years, it has also proved to be useful to adults. Or, used in conjunction with a keto diet, certain people with epilepsy might be able to take less to no anti-epileptic drugs while being seizure-free. This may help to reduce the drug's adverse effects while still improving cognitive capacity.

Keto Chaffle Recipes

1 Oreo Chaffles

(Ready in about 23 minutes | Serving 2 | Difficulty: Easy)

Per serving: Kcal 1381, Fat: 146g, Net Carbs: 14g, Protein: 17g

Ingredients

- 1/2 cup of Sugar-Free Chocolate Chips
- 1 tsp of Vanilla extract
- 3 Eggs
- 1/2 cup of butter
- 1/4 cup of sweetener

Cheese Frosting

- 4 ounces of Cream Cheese
- 4 ounces of butter
- 1/2 cup of Powdered Swerve
- 1 tsp of Vanilla extract
- 1/4 cup of Whipping Cream

Instructions

Melt chocolate and butter in a bowl in the microwave for around 1 minute. Stir remove clumps. Mix vanilla, egg and sweetener in a bowl. Pour a quarter of t mixture into the waffle maker and cook for around 8 minutes. Mix frosting ingredien in the food processor's bowl in the meantime and make a smooth mixture. Spre frosting among two chaffles.

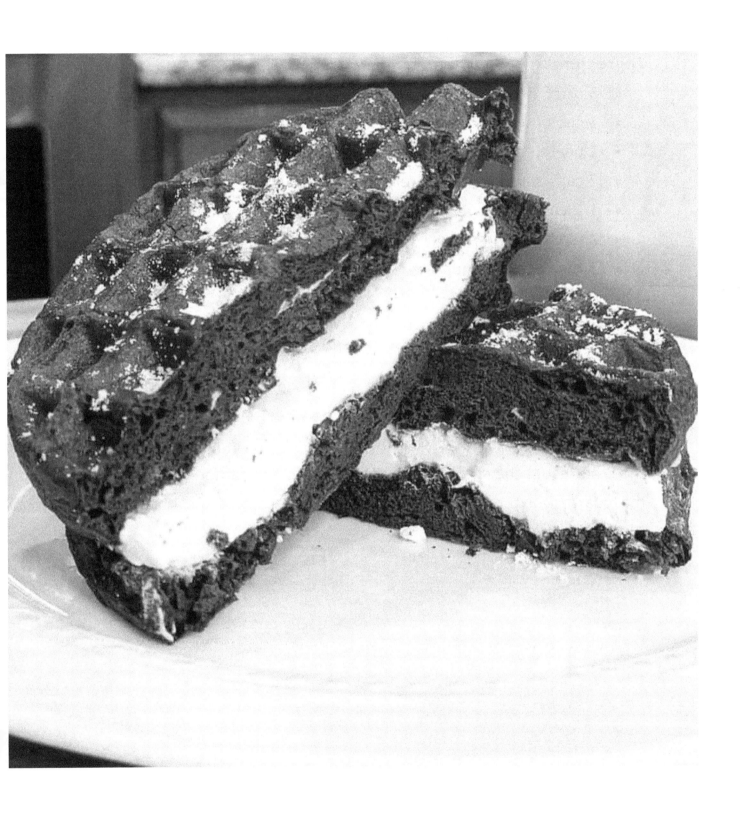

2 Strawberry Chaffles

(Ready in about 35 minutes | Serving 8 | Difficulty: Moderate)

Per serving: Kcal 189, Fat: 14.3g, Net Carbs: 5.2g, Protein: 10g

Ingredients

- 3 oz of cream cheese
- 1 cup of whipped cream
- 2 beaten eggs
- 2 cups shredded mozzarella cheese
- 1/2 cup of almond flour
- 2 tsp of baking powder
- 3 tbsp of sweetener
- 8 strawberries
- 1 tbsp of sweetener

Instructions

Add mozzarella and cream cheese to a bowl and microwave for around 1 minute. Be
eggs and mix with baking powder, 3 tbsp sweetener and almond flour. Mix it w
cheese and add to 2 diced strawberries. Place in the fridge for around 20 minute
Dice the rest of the strawberries and add tbsp sweetener. Warm waffle iron and a
the quarter mixture from the fridge to the center of the iron. Cook for around
minutes.

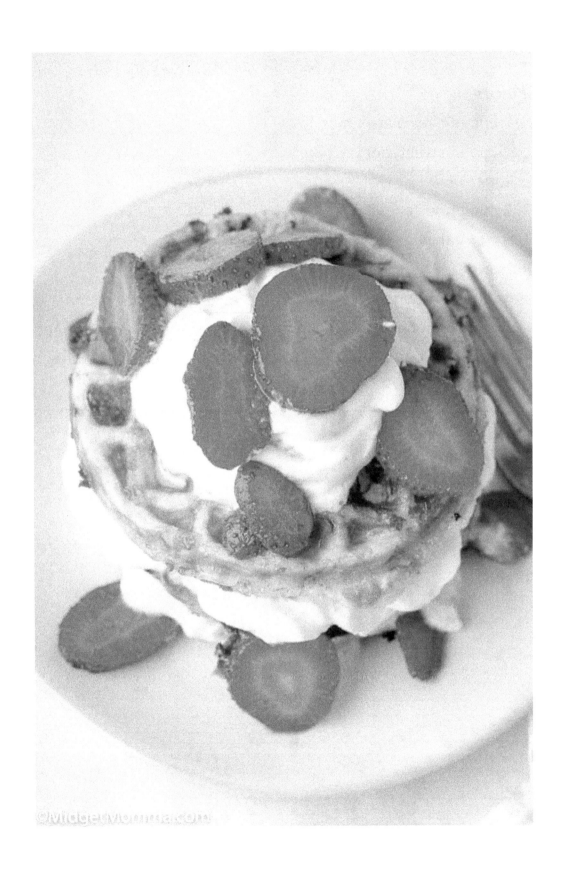

3 Chocolate Chaffle

(Ready in about 18 minutes | Serving 2 | Difficulty: Easy)

Per serving: Kcal 672, Fat: 70g, Net Carbs: 11g, Protein: 13g

Ingredients

- 1/2 cup of Chocolate Chips
- 1/4 cup of sweetener
- 3 Eggs
- 1/2 cup of butter
- 1 tsp of Vanilla extract

Instructions

Melt chocolate and butter in a bowl in the microwave for around 1 minute. Stir ar remove clumps. Blend sweetener, vanilla and eggs in a bowl. Add chocolate an butter and whisk. Pour the quarter amount of mixture into a waffle maker. Cook f around 8 minutes.

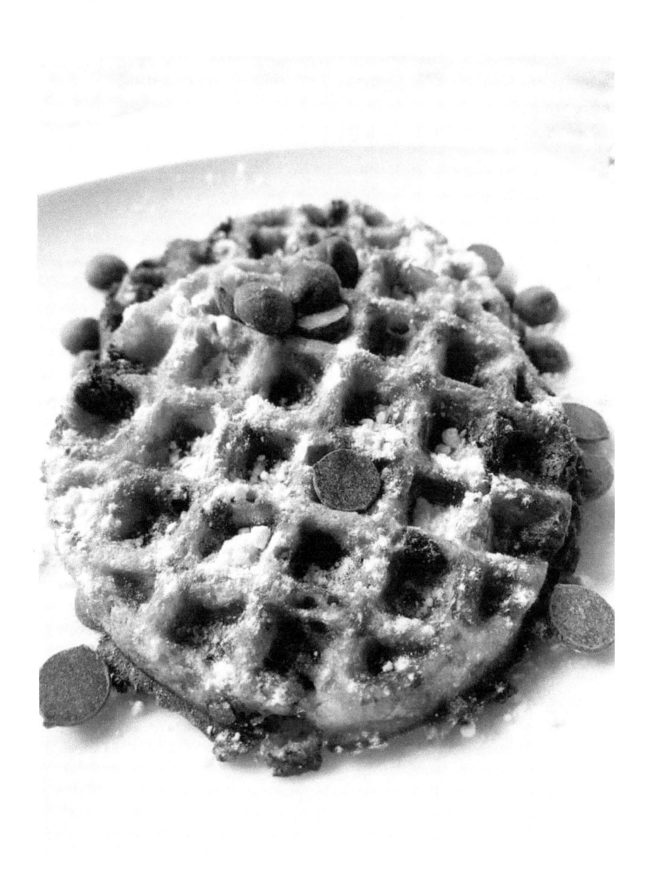

4 Pumpkin Chaffles

(Ready in about 7 minutes | Serving 1 | Difficulty: Easy)

Per serving: Kcal 250, Fat: 15g, Net Carbs: 5g, Protein: 23g

Ingredients

- 1/2 cup mozzarella cheese shredded
- 1 1/2tbsp of pumpkin purée
- 1 beaten egg
- 1/2tsp of Swerve confectioners
- 1/4tsp of Pumpkin Pie Spice
- 1/2tsp of vanilla extract
- ⅛ tsp of maple extract

Instructions

Mix all the ingredients except mozzarella cheese in a bowl and mix. Add cheese a whisk. Spray waffle using cooking spray. Place half amount of batter in the center the waffle maker. Cook for around 6 minutes. Repeat with the remaining batter.

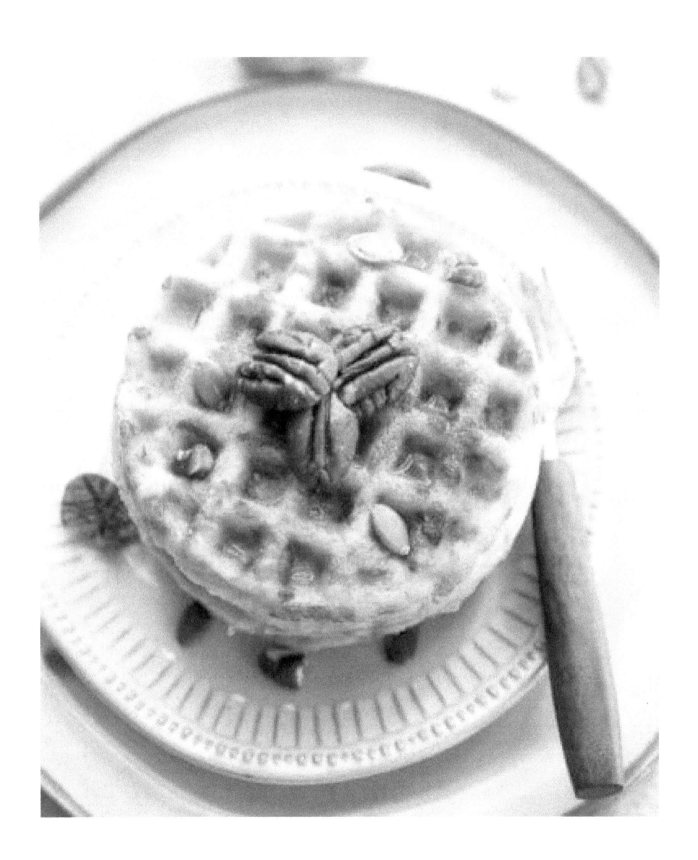

5 Basic Chaffle

(Ready in about 8 minutes | Serving 2 | Difficulty: Easy)

Per serving: Kcal 208, Fat: 16g, Net Carbs: 4g, Protein: 11g

Ingredients

- 1 Big Egg
- 2 tbsp of Almond Flour
- 1/2 cup shredded Mozzarella cheese

Instructions

Preheat waffle iron for around 5 minutes. Microwave cheese for around 30 second
Add the rest of the ingredients and mix. Pour mixture that covers the surface of th
waffle maker. Cook for around 4 minutes. Take out and place on a plate and repe
with the rest of the batter.

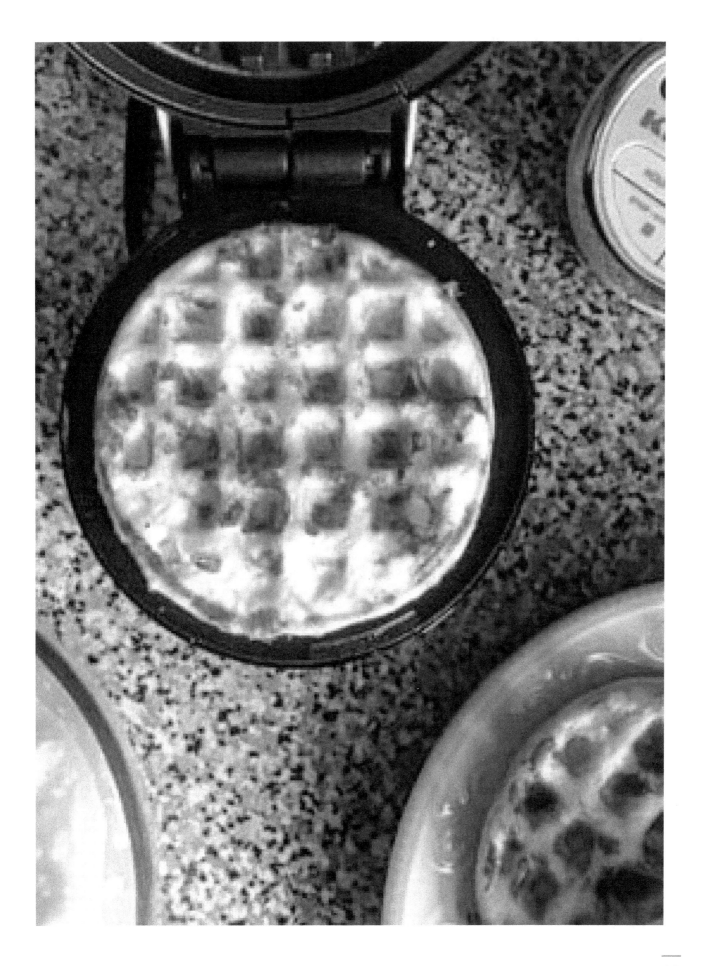

6 Garlic Chaffles

(Ready in about 8 minutes | Serving 2 | Difficulty: Easy)

Per serving: Kcal 208, Fat: 16g, Net Carbs: 4g, Protein: 11g

Ingredients

- 1/3 cup Parmesan cheese Grated
- 1/2 cup shredded Mozzarella cheese
- 1 Big Egg
- 1/2 tsp of Italian seasoning
- 1 minced Garlic clove

Instructions

Preheat waffle iron for around 5 minutes. Microwave cream cheese for around seconds. Add the rest of the ingredients except the toppings. Pour mixture that cove the surface of the waffle maker. Cook for around 4 minutes. Take out and place or plate and repeat with the rest of the batter.

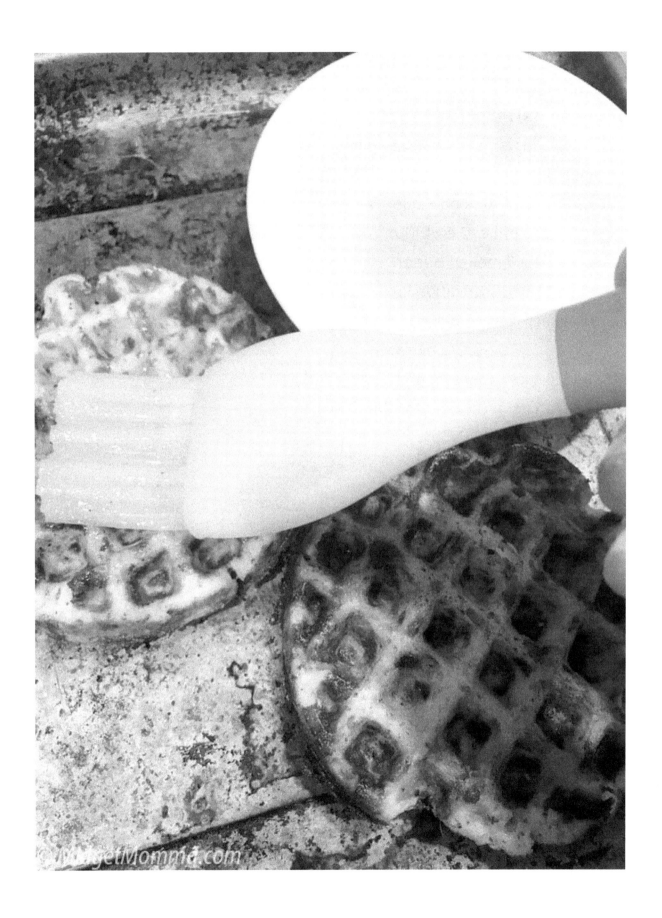

©BudgetMomma.com

7 Cinnamon Chaffles

(Ready in about 8 minutes | Serving 2 | Difficulty: Easy)

Per serving: Kcal 208, Fat: 16g, Net Carbs: 4g, Protein: 11g

Ingredients

- 3/4 cup shredded Mozzarella cheese
- 1 Big Egg
- 2 tbsp of Almond Flour
- 2 tbsp of besti erythritol
- 1/2 tbsp melted butter
- 1/2 tsp of cinnamon
- 1 tbsp melted butter
- 1/2 tsp of vanilla extract
- 3/4 tsp of cinnamon
- 1/4 cup of besti erythritol

Instructions

Preheat waffle iron for around 5 minutes. Microwave cream cheese for around 30 seconds. Add the rest of the ingredients except the toppings. Pour mixture that covers the surface of the waffle maker. Cook for around 4 minutes. Take out and place on a plate and repeat with the rest of the batter. To prepare churro chaffles, mix cinnamon and erythritol for topping. Brush chaffles using butter after they are cooked and sprinkle with topping.

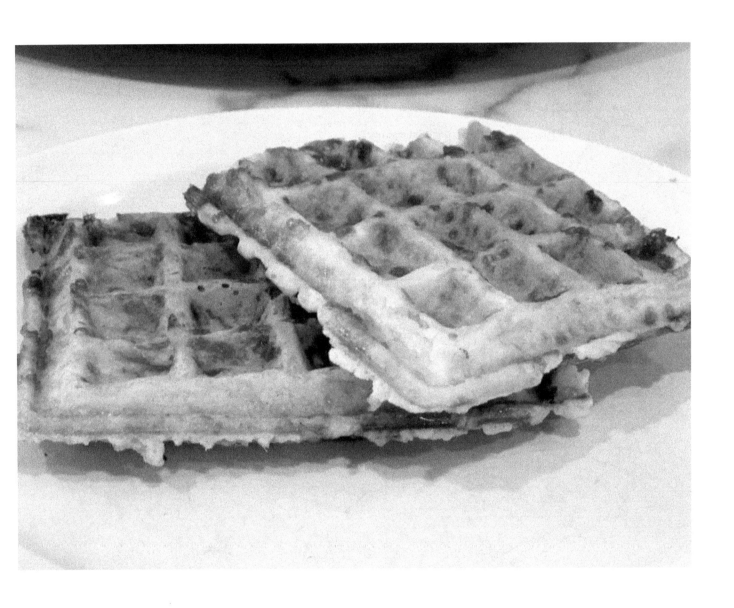

8 Cheese Chaffles

(Ready in about 8 minutes | Serving 2 | Difficulty: Easy)

Per serving: Kcal 208, Fat: 16g, Net Carbs: 4g, Protein: 11g

Ingredients

- 1 Egg
- 1/2 oz of Cream cheese
- 1/2 cup shredded Mozzarella cheese
- 2 1/2 tbsp of Besti Erythritol
- 2 tbsp of pumpkin puree
- 1/2 tbsp of Pumpkin pie spice
- 3 tsp of Coconut Flour

Instructions

Preheat waffle iron for around 5 minutes. Microwave cream cheese for around seconds. Add the rest of the ingredients except the toppings. Pour mixture that cove the surface of the waffle maker. Cook for around 4 minutes. Take out and place or plate and repeat with the rest of the batter.

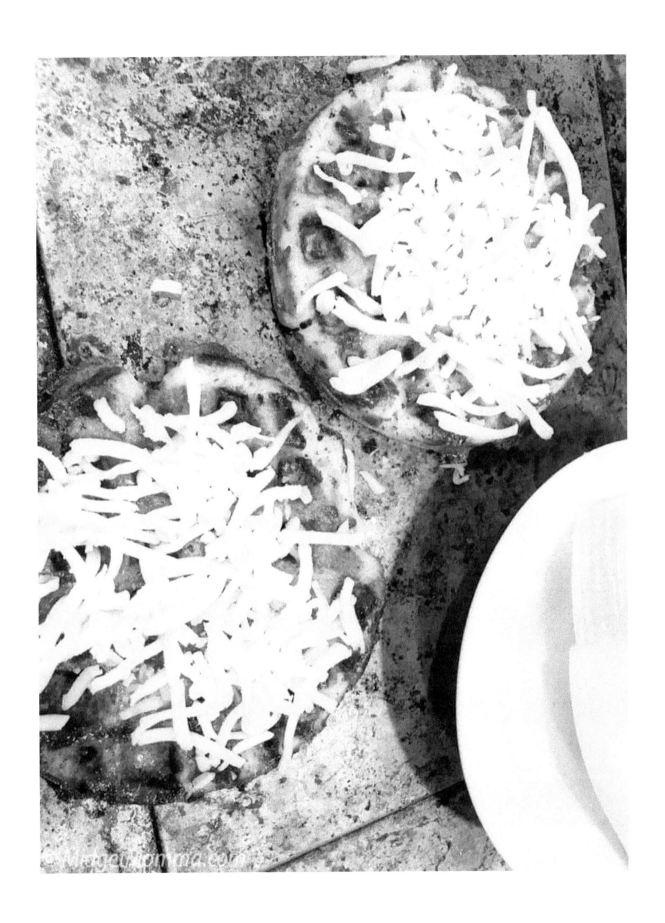

9 Spicy Chaffles

(Ready in about 8 minutes | Serving 2 | Difficulty: Easy)

Per serving: Kcal 208, Fat: 16g, Net Carbs: 4g, Protein: 11g

Ingredients

- 1 Egg
- 1 oz of Cream cheese
- 1 cup shredded Cheddar cheese
- 1/2 tbsp of Jalapenos
- 2 tbsp of Bacon bits

Instructions

Preheat waffle iron for around 5 minutes. Microwave cream cheese for around seconds. Add the rest of the ingredients except the toppings. Pour mixture that cove the surface of the waffle maker. Cook for around 4 minutes. Take out and place on plate and repeat with the rest of the batter.

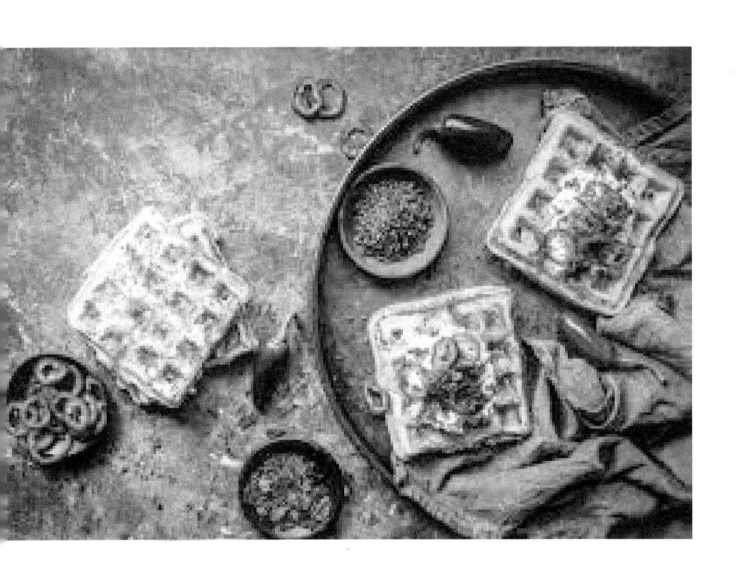

10 Double Chocolate Chaffles

(Ready in about 5 minutes | Serving 1 | Difficulty: Easy)

Per serving: Kcal 197, Fat: 23.3g, Net Carbs: 11.3g, Protein: 24.3g

Ingredients

- 1 egg
- 1 tbsp of granulated sweetener
- 1/2 cup grated mozzarella
- 1 tsp of vanilla
- 1 tbsp of chocolate chips
- 2 tbsp of almond meal/flour
- 1 tsp of heavy cream
- 2 tbsp unsweetened cocoa powder

Instructions

Add all the ingredients to a bowl and mix. Preheat the waffle maker. Spray with
and pour half amount of batter into the maker. Cook for around 4 minutes. Sprinl
with toppings and enjoy.

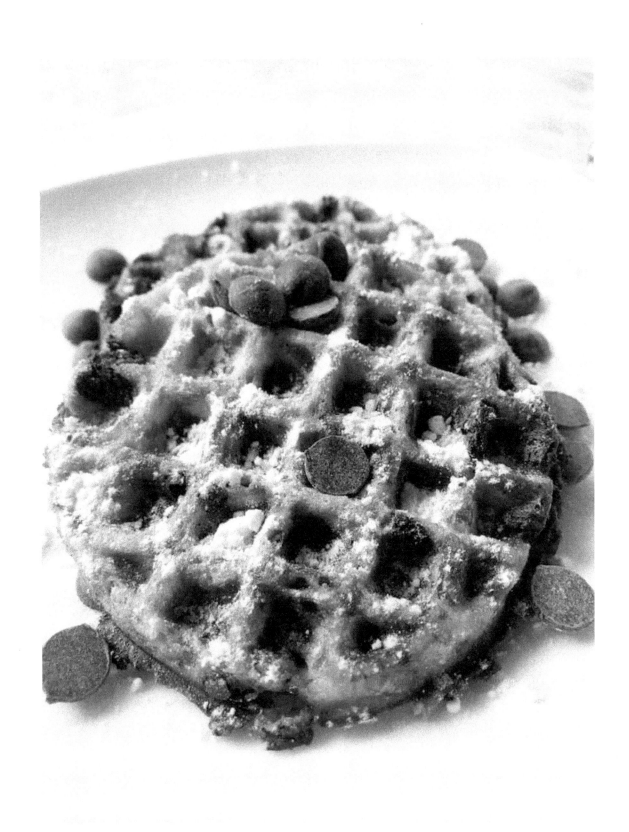

11 Vanilla Chaffles

(Ready in about 10 minutes | Serving 1 | Difficulty: Easy)

Per serving: Kcal 184, Fat: 20.1g, Net Carbs: 5.4g, Protein: 22.2g

Ingredients

- 1/2 cup of grated mozzarella
- 1 tbsp of granulated sweetener
- 1 eggs
- 1 tsp of vanilla extract
- 1 tbsp of chocolate chips
- 2 tbsp of almond flour

Instructions

Combine all the ingredients in a bowl. Preheat the waffle maker and spray it using once it is hot. Pour half amount of batter in the maker and cook for around 4 minute Remove and do the same with the rest of the batter. Top and enjoy.

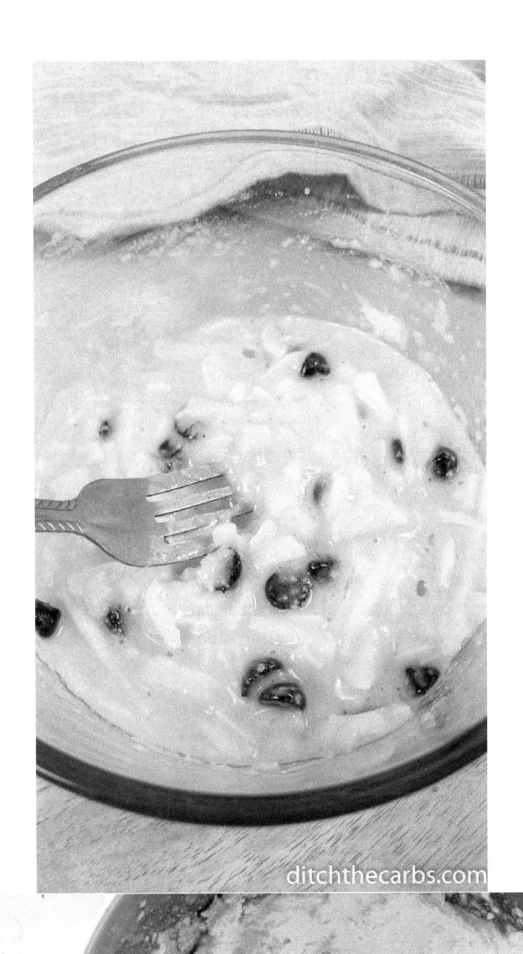

12 Lemon Curd Chaffle

(Ready in about 50 minutes | Serving 3 | Difficulty: Hard)

Per serving: Kcal 302, Fat: 24g, Net Carbs: 6g, Protein: 15g

Ingredients

- 3 eggs
- one batch of lemon curd
- 4 ounces softened cream cheese
- 1 tsp of vanilla extract
- 1 tbsp sweetener low carb
- 3/4 cup shredded mozzarella cheese
- 1 tsp of baking powder
- 3 tbsp of coconut flour
- 1/3 tsp of salt

Instructions

Prepare lemon curd according to package instructions. Heat the maker and spray c
Mix baking powder, salt and coconut flour in a bowl. Add the rest of the ingredier
to another bowl and beat using a hand blender. Mix the two bowls mixture and po
in the maker. Cook for around 5 minutes. Top using lemon curd.

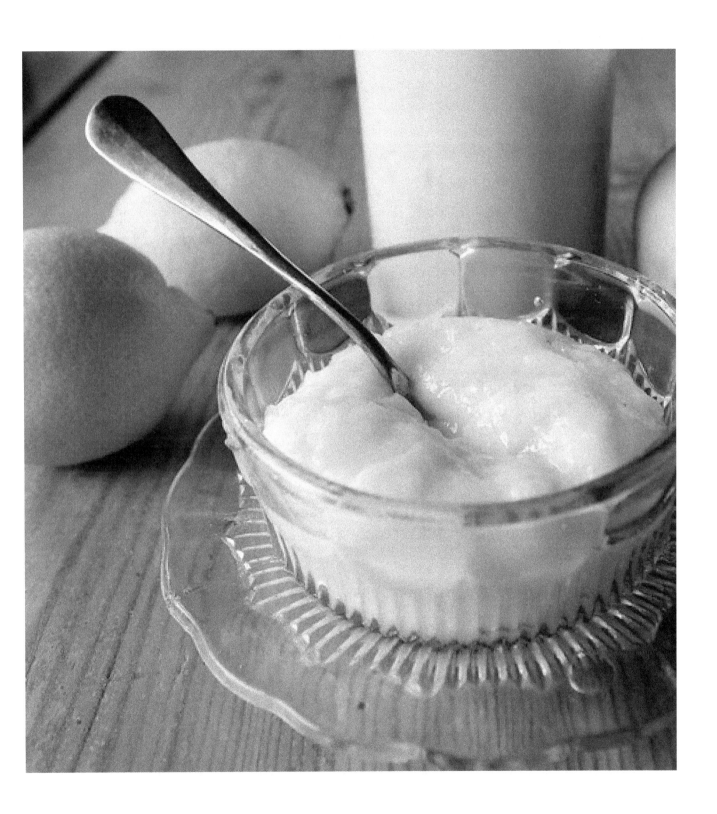

13 Glazed Donut

(Ready in about 15 minutes | Serving 3 | Difficulty: Easy)

Per serving: Kcal 246, Fat: 17g, Net Carbs: 2g, Protein: 14g

Ingredients

For chaffles

- 1/2 cup shredded cheese Mozzarella
- 2 tbsp of whey protein
- 1 ounce of Cream Cheese
- 2 tbsp of Swerve confectioners
- 1/2tsp of Vanilla extract
- 1/2tsp of Baking powder
- 1 Egg

For glaze

- 1/2tsp of Vanilla extract
- 3-4 tbsp of Swerve confectioners
- 2 tbsp of whipping cream

Instructions

Preheat the waffle maker. Add cream cheese and mozzarella in a bowl and microwave for around 30 seconds. Add 2 tbsp sweetener, whey protein and baking powder and mix. Add dough to a bowl and break an egg into it and add vanilla. Stir to form smooth mixture. Add batter to the waffle maker and cook for around 5 minutes. Beat glaze ingredients in a bowl and top chaffles with it.

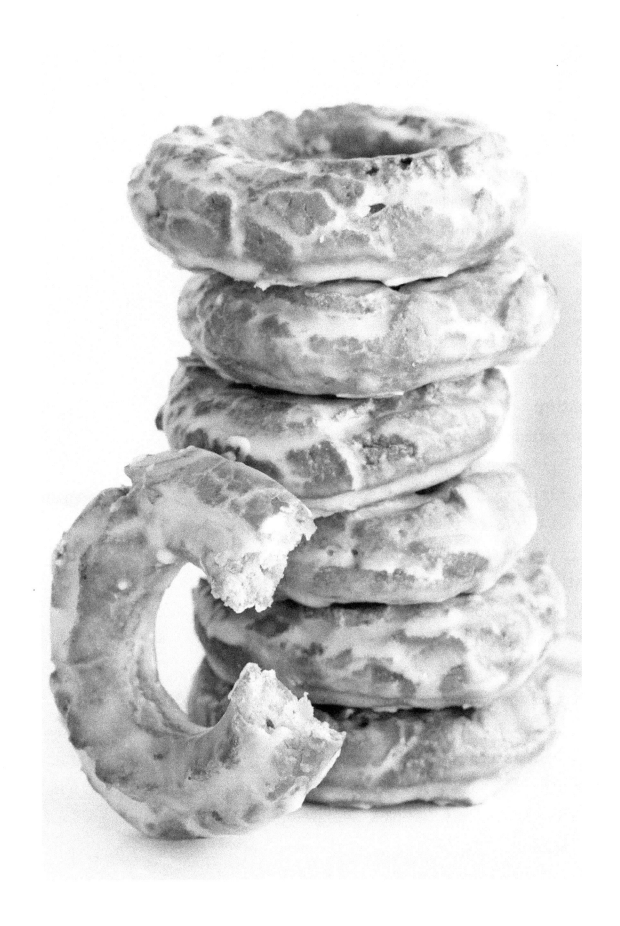

14 Nut-Free Chaffles

(Ready in about 30 minutes | Serving 3 | Difficulty: Easy)

Per serving: Kcal 195, Fat: 15.1g, Net Carbs: 31.5g, Protein: 8.5g

Ingredients

Batter

- 1/2 cup shredded cheese mozzarella
- 1/4 tsp of vanilla extract
- 2 tbsp of SunButter
- 2 tbsp of fruit sweetener
- 1 egg
- 2 tsp of cinnamon
- 1 tbsp of coconut flour
- ⅛ tsp of baking powder

Frosting

- 1 tbsp of cream cheese
- 1/4 cup of fruit sweetener
- 3/4 tbsp of butter, melted
- 1 tbsp of coconut milk unsweetened
- 1/4 tsp of vanilla extract

Coating

- 1 tsp of fruit sweetener
- 1 tsp of cinnamon

Instructions

Preheat the waffle iron. Mix batter ingredients in a bowl and place aside. Mix frosti
ingredients except for coconut milk in a bowl and whisk until smooth. Add cocor
milk and mix again. Place aside. Coat iron with cooking spray and add batter. Co
for around 4 minutes. Sprinkle with sweetener and cinnamon.

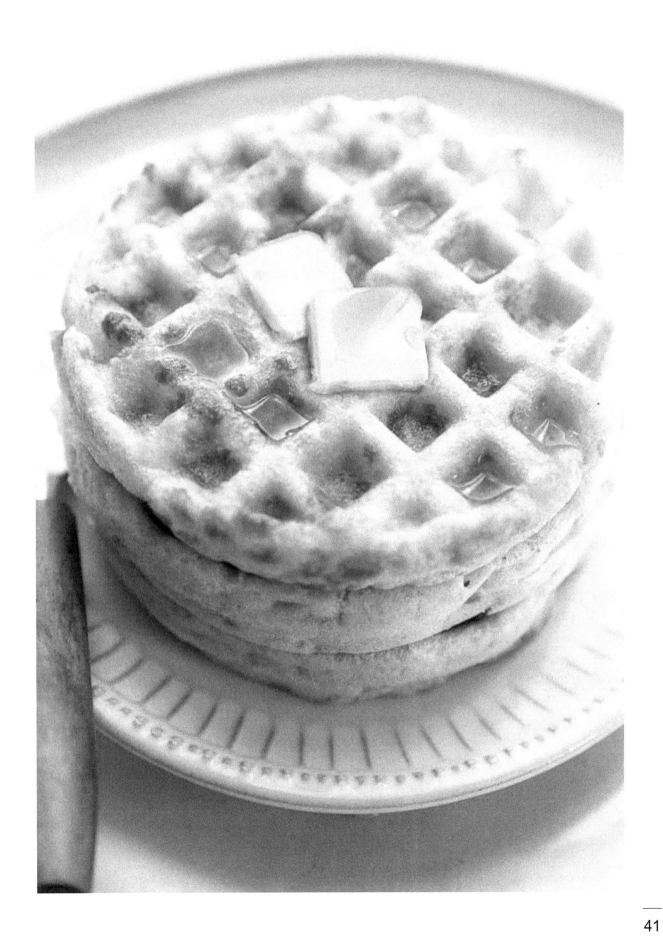

15 Chicken Chaffle

(Ready in about 19 minutes | Serving 2 | Difficulty: Easy)

Per serving: Kcal 675, Fat: 52g, Net Carbs: 8g, Protein: 44g

Ingredients

- 1/4 cup of almond flour
- 1/4 cup crumbled feta cheese
- 2 eggs
- 1 tsp of baking powder
- 1/2 cup shredded chicken
- 1/4 cup of Hot Sauce
- 1/4 cup shredded mozzarella cheese
- 3/4 cup shredded cheddar cheese
- 1/4 cup diced celery

Instructions

Mix almond flour and baking powder in a bowl. Preheat iron and spray using cooking spray. Beat eggs in a bowl and add hot sauce. Combine thoroughly and pour flour mixture. Combine and add grated cheeses. Fold in chicken. Pour in the maker and cook for around 4 minutes. Top with celery and feta.

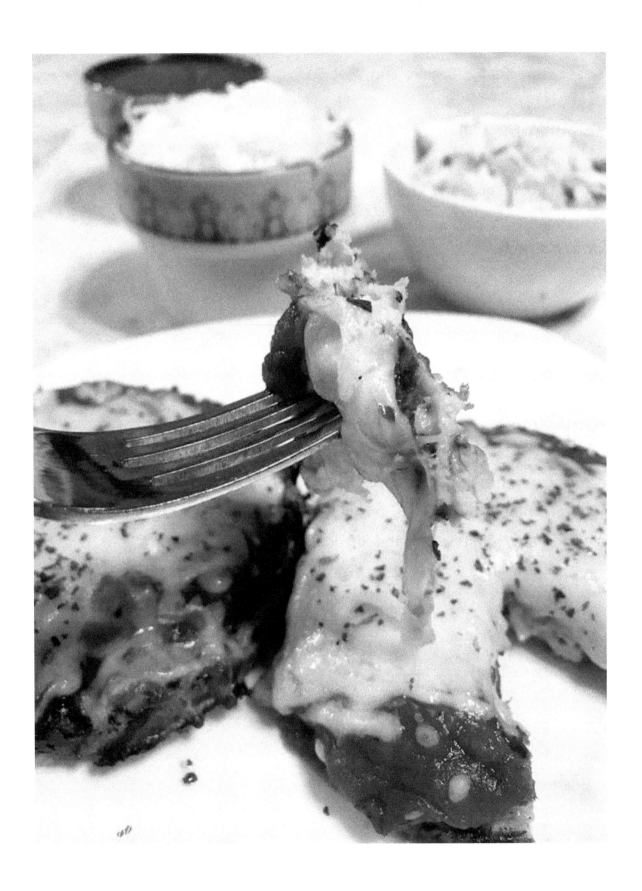

16 Chaffle Sandwich

(Ready in about 13 minutes | Serving 1 | Difficulty: Easy)

Per serving: Kcal 238, Fat: 18g, Net Carbs: 2g, Protein: 17g

Ingredients

For chaffles

- 1/2 cup shredded Cheddar cheese
- 1 egg

For sandwich

- 1 tbsp of mayonnaise
- 2 slices of tomato
- 2 strips of bacon
- 3 pieces of lettuce

Instructions

Preheat the maker and mix cheese and egg in a bowl. Pour batter into the maker a cook for around 4 minutes. Do it in 2 batches. Cook bacon in pan paced on t moderate flame until it gets crispy. Drain using paper towels and form a sandwi using tomato, mayonnaise and lettuce.

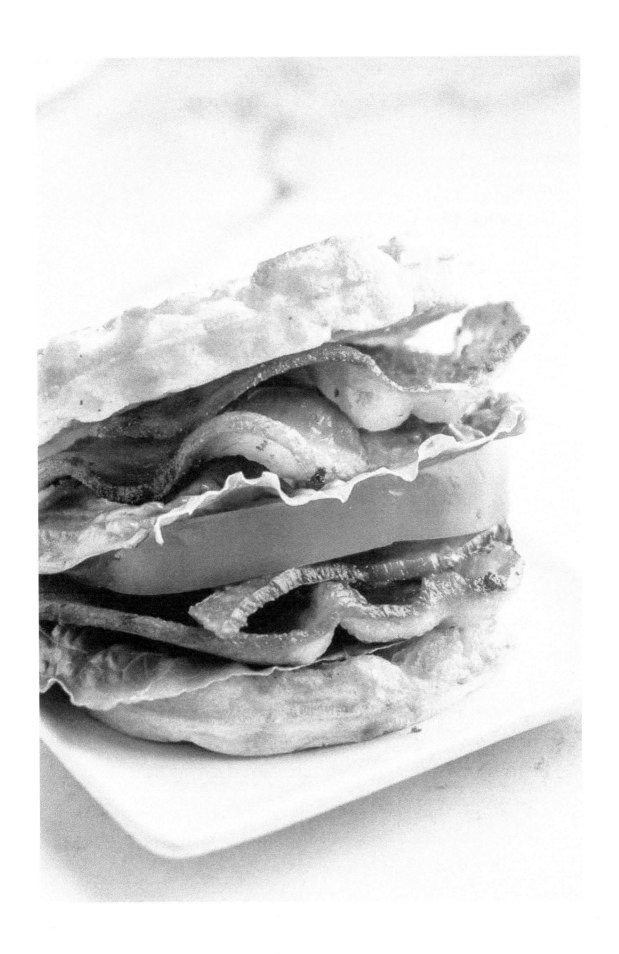

17 Sausage Gravy Chaffle

(Ready in about 15 minutes | Serving 2 | Difficulty: Easy)

Per serving: Kcal 212, Fat: 17g, Net Carbs: 3g, Protein: 11g

Ingredients

For Chaffle

- 1/2 cup grated mozzarella cheese
- 1 egg
- 1 tsp of coconut flour
- 1/4 tsp of baking powder
- 1 tsp of water
- Salt

For Gravy

- 3 tbsp of chicken broth
- 1/4 cup browned breakfast sausage
- 2 tbsp of whipping cream
- dash of garlic powder
- 2 tsp softened cream cheese
- pepper

Instructions

Preheat the maker and coat using cooking spray. Add all ingredients to a bowl a mix. Pour half amount to mixture into the maker and cook for around 4 minute Repeat with the remaining batter and enjoy. Prepare breakfast sausage and add the pan with remaining ingredients and boil. Reduce flame and cook for around minutes to thicken it. Add pepper and salt and spoon gravy on top of chaffles.

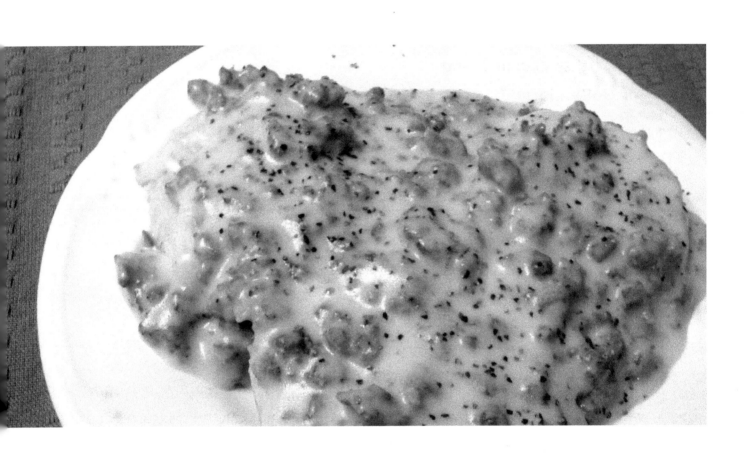

18 Eggs Benedict

(Ready in about 30 minutes | Serving 2 | Difficulty: Easy)

Per serving: Kcal 844, Fat: 78g, Net Carbs: 5g, Protein: 32g

Ingredients

For Chaffles

- 1/2 cup of mozzarella cheese
- 2 tbsp of almond flour
- 2 whites of eggs
- 1 tbsp of sour cream

For Hollandaise

- 2 tbsp of lemon juice
- 4 yolks of eggs
- 1/2 cup of salted butter

For Eggs

- 1 tbsp of white vinegar
- 3 ounces of deli ham
- 2 eggs

Instructions

Whisk eggs in a bowl and with the rest of the ingredients and blend. Preheat t waffle maker. Spray using cooking spray and add half the mixture. Cook for arou 7 minutes. Make hollandaise sauce by forming a double broiler. Boil water and wa butter in the microwave. Add egg to bowl of the boiler. Boil and add hot butter wh the pot is carried to a boil. Cook until egg thickens and take out of the bowl. Driz lemon juice and place aside. Warm chaffle using toaster and top with ham slices, tbsp hollandaise sauce and one egg.

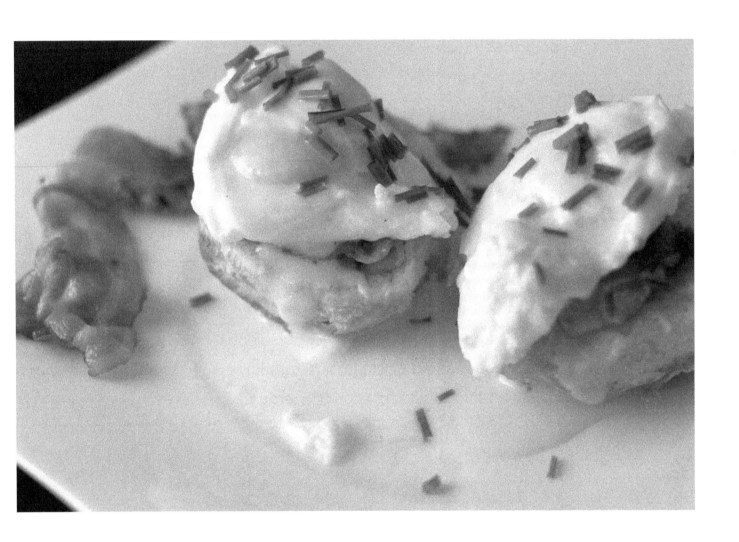

19 Garlic Chaffle

(Ready in about 10 minutes | Serving 8 | Difficulty: Easy)

Per serving: Kcal 74, Fat: 6.5g, Net Carbs: 0.9g, Protein: 3.4g

Ingredients

- 1 egg
- 2 tbsp of almond flour
- 1/2 cup grated mozzarella cheese
- 1/2tsp of garlic powder
- 1/2tsp of salt
- 1/2tsp of oregano

Topping

- 1/2tsp of garlic powder
- 2 tbsp softened butter
- 1/4 cup grated mozzarella cheese

Instructions

Preheat the maker and oil it. Mix ingredients except topping ingredients. Pour in the maker and cook for around 5 minutes. Mix garlic powder and butter and pour ov waffle. Sprinkle with mozzarella and cook for around 3 minutes.

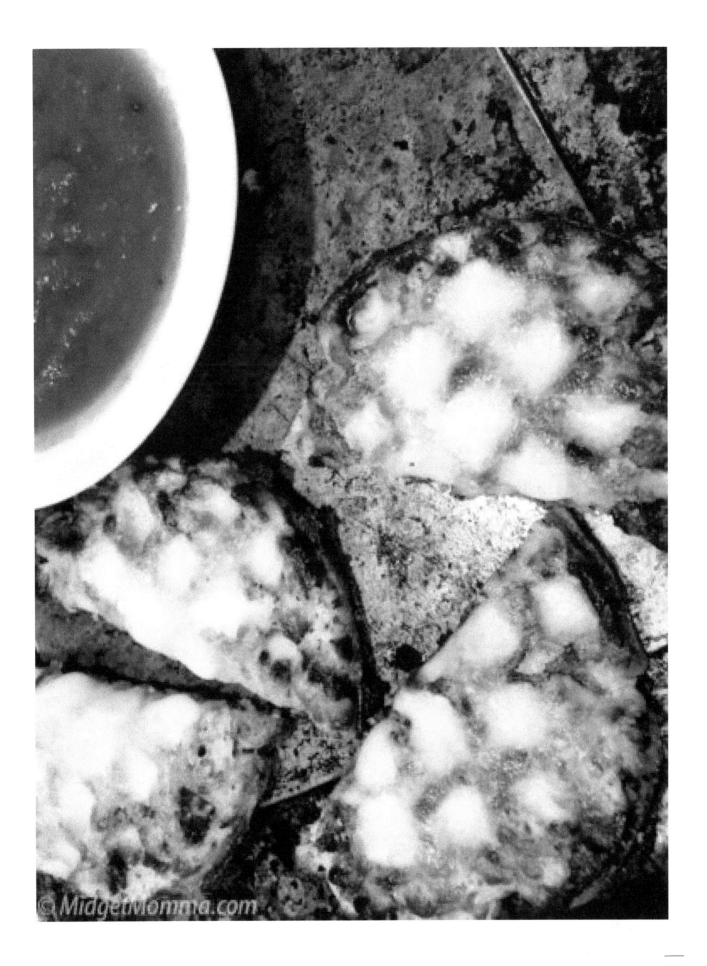

20 Taco Chaffle

(Ready in about 13 minutes | Serving 1 | Difficulty: Easy)

Per serving: Kcal 258, Fat: 19g, Net Carbs: 4g, Protein: 18g

Ingredients

- 1/4 cup shredded jack cheese
- 1 white of egg
- 1/4 cup shredded cheddar cheese
- 1 tsp of coconut flour
- 3/4 tsp of water
- 1/4 tsp of baking powder
- pinch of salt
- 1/8 tsp of chili powder

Instructions

Preheat the maker and oil it. Combine everything in a bowl and spoon half amount mixture in the maker. Cook for around 4 minutes. Remove the chaffle shell and pla it aside. Repeat with the remaining batter. Turn the pan and position shells of t chaffle among cups to make a shell of taco.

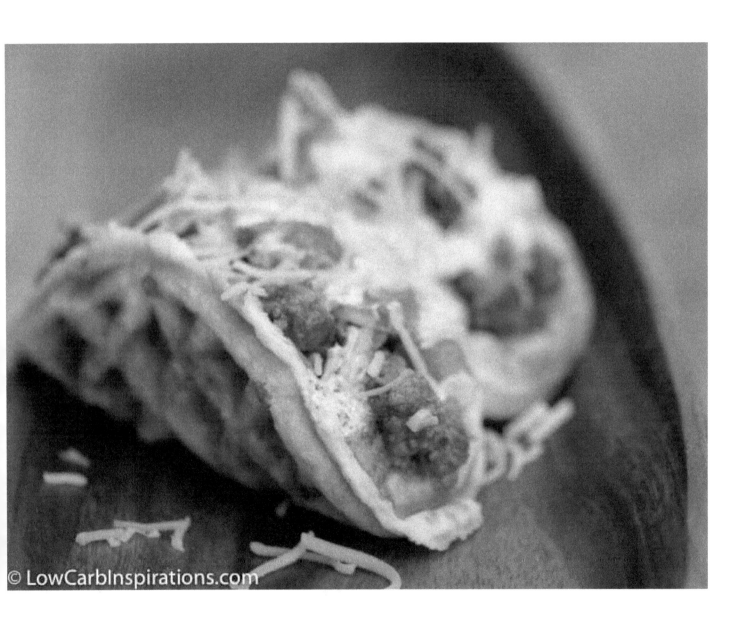

21 Pizza Chaffle

(Ready in about 8 minutes | Serving 2 | Difficulty: Easy)

Per serving: Kcal 76, Fat: 4.3g, Net Carbs: 4.1g, Protein: 5.5g

Ingredients

- 1 egg
- Pinch of Italian seasoning
- 1/2 cup shredded mozzarella cheese
- 1 tbsp of pizza sauce

Instructions

Preheat the maker. Whisk eggs in a bowl and add seasonings. Mix shredded chees in a bowl. Add half amount of mixture to the maker and cook for around 4 minute Repeat with the rest of the batter and with 1 tbsp pizza sauce and pepperoni.

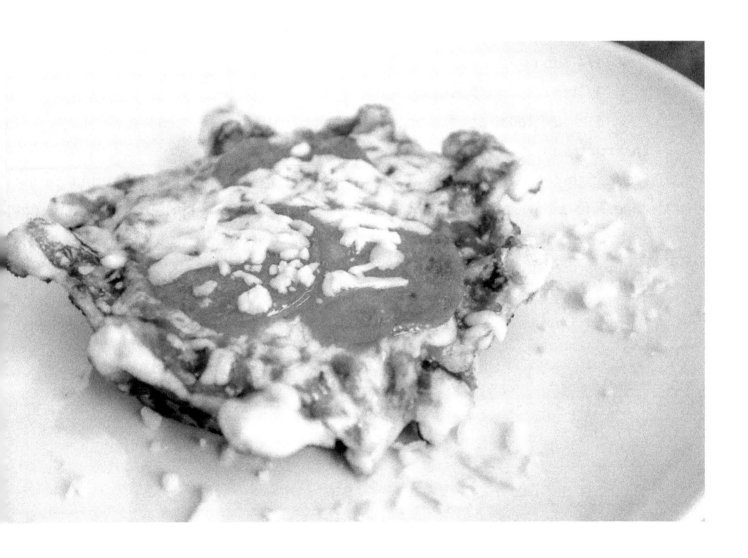

22 Parmesan Chaffles

(Ready in about 6 minutes | Serving 1 | Difficulty: Easy)

Per serving: Kcal 352, Fat: 24g, Net Carbs: 2g, Protein: 14g

Ingredients

- 1 beaten egg
- 1/2 cup of mozzarella cheese shredded
- 1/4 cup of Parmesan cheese grated
- 1/4tsp of garlic powder
- 1 tsp of Italian seasoning

Instructions

Preheat the waffle maker. Add all the ingredients except mozzarella and parmes
cheese in a bowl and mix. Mix the cheese in a bowl and spray waffle sung cooki
spray. Pour half amount of mixture in the maker and cook for around 5 minutes. T
using parmesan and enjoy.

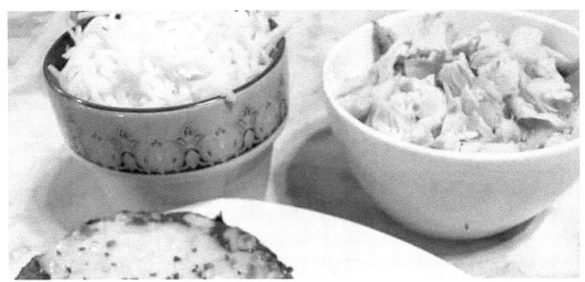

CHICKEN PARMESAN Chaffle

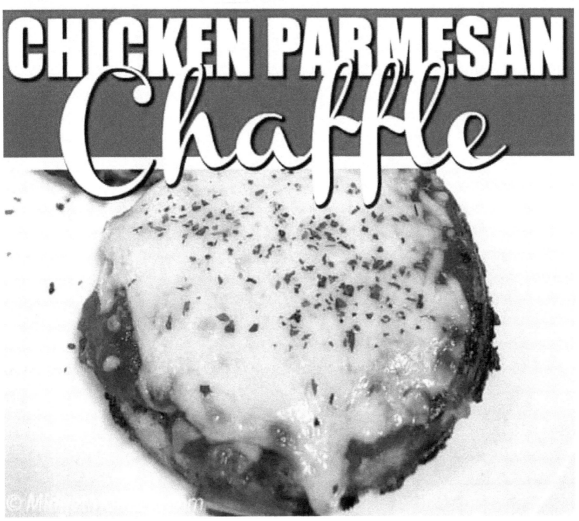

23 Italian Chaffle

(Ready in about 6 minutes | Serving 1 | Difficulty: Easy)

Per serving: Kcal 352, Fat: 24g, Net Carbs: 2g, Protein: 14g

Ingredients

- 1 beaten egg
- 1/2 cup of mozzarella cheese shredded
- 1/4 cup of Parmesan cheese grated
- 1/4tsp of garlic powder
- 1 tsp of Italian seasoning

Instructions

Preheat the waffle maker. Add all the ingredients except mozzarella and parmesa cheese in a bowl and mix. Mix the cheese in a bowl and spray waffle sung cookir spray. Pour half amount of mixture in the maker and cook for around 5 minutes. To using parmesan and add lettuce, cold cuts, tomato.

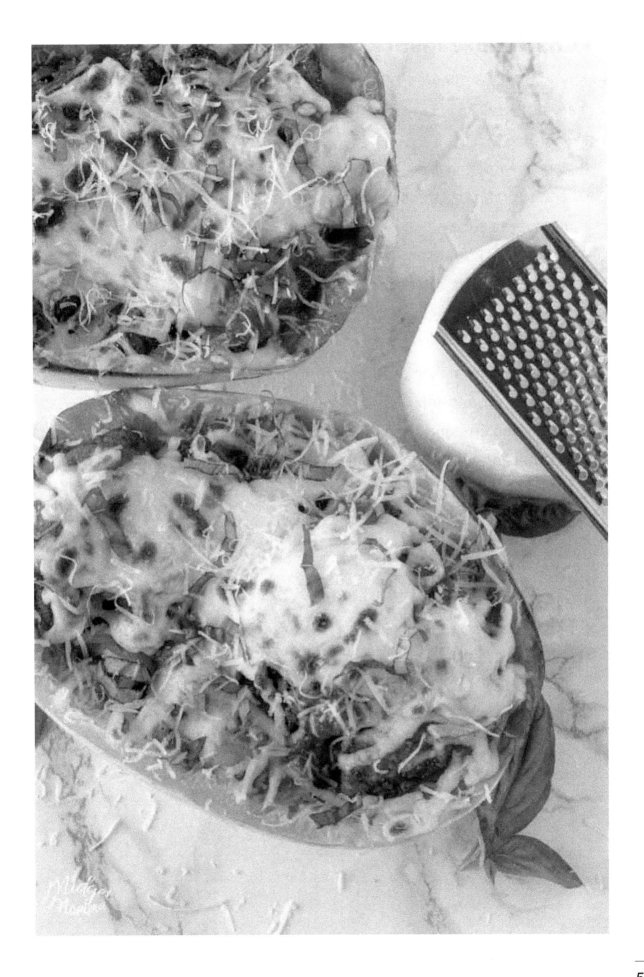

24 Chaffle Breadsticks

(Ready in about 6 minutes | Serving 1 | Difficulty: Easy)

Per serving: Kcal 352, Fat: 24g, Net Carbs: 2g, Protein: 14g

Ingredients

- 1 beaten egg
- 1/2 cup of mozzarella cheese shredded
- Marinara sauce
- 1/4 cup of Parmesan cheese grated
- 1/4tsp of garlic powder
- 1 tsp of Italian seasoning

Instructions

Preheat the waffle maker. Add all the ingredients except mozzarella and parmes
cheese in a bowl and mix. Mix the cheese in a bowl and spray waffle sung cooki
spray. Pour half amount of mixture in the maker and cook for around 5 minutes. T
using parmesan and dice into 4 sticks and enjoy with Marinara Sauce.

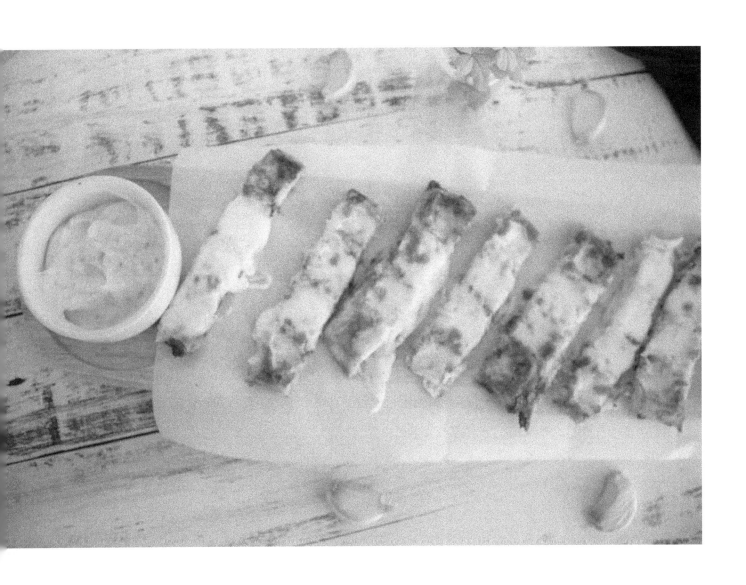

25 Chaffle Bruschetta

(Ready in about 6 minutes | Serving 1 | Difficulty: Easy)

Per serving: Kcal 352, Fat: 24g, Net Carbs: 2g, Protein: 14g

Ingredients

- 1 beaten egg
- 1/2 cup of mozzarella cheese shredded
- 1/4 cup of Parmesan cheese grated
- Basil
- Olive oil
- 1/4tsp of garlic powder
- 1 tsp of Italian seasoning

Instructions

Preheat the waffle maker. Add all the ingredients except mozzarella and parmesa cheese in a bowl and mix. Mix the cheese in a bowl and spray waffle sung cookir spray. Pour half amount of mixture in the maker and cook for around 5 minutes. T using parmesan and mix 4 chopped cherry tomatoes, ½ tsp chopped fresh basil, drc of olive oil and salt. Add on chaffle.

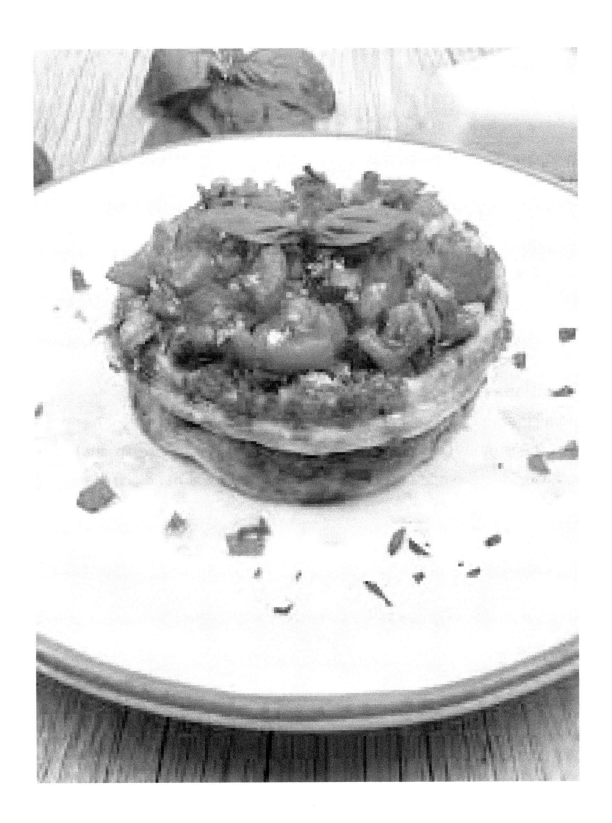

26 Cauliflower Chaffles

(Ready in about 9 minutes | Serving 2 | Difficulty: Easy)

Per serving: Kcal 246, Fat: 16g, Net Carbs: 7g, Protein: 20g

Ingredients

- 1/4 tsp of Garlic Powder
- 1 cup of riced cauliflower
- 1/4 tsp of Ground Black Pepper
- 1/4 tsp of Kosher Salt
- 1/2 tsp of Italian seasoning
- 1 Eggs
- 1/2 cup of mozzarella cheese shredded
- 1/2 cup of parmesan cheese shredded

Instructions

Blend all ingredients except the cauliflower mixture and parmesan cheese in a blend and sprinkle half parmesan in the maker. Pour mixture in maker and top wi cauliflower mixture and rest of parmesan. Cook for around 5 minutes.

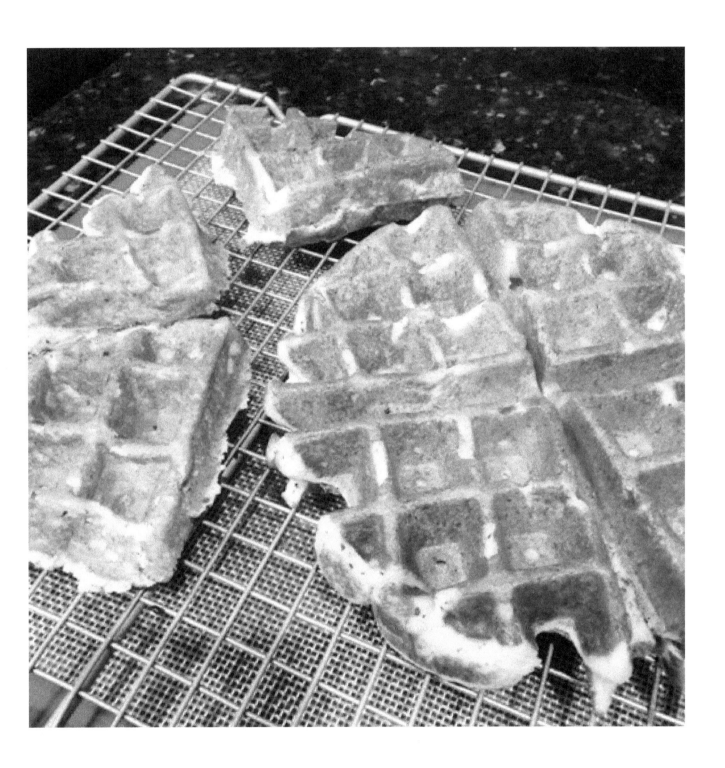

27 Zucchini Chaffles

(Ready in about 15 minutes | Serving 2 | Difficulty: Easy)

Per serving: Kcal 194, Fat: 13g, Net Carbs: 4g, Protein: 16g

Ingredients

- 1 beaten Egg
- 1/2 tsp Black Pepper Ground
- 1 cup grated Zucchini
- 1/2 cup of parmesan cheese shredded
- 1 tsp chopped Dried Basil
- 1/4 cup of mozzarella cheese shredded
- 3/4 tsp divided Kosher Salt

Instructions

Sprinkle 1/4 tsp salt on zucchini. Beat egg in a bowl and add mozzarella, zucchin 1/2 tsp salt, basil and pepper. Sprinkle 2 tbsp parmesan on iron and spread a quart of zucchini mixture on the maker. Top using 2 tbsp parmesan and cook for around minutes. Repeat with the rest of the mixture.

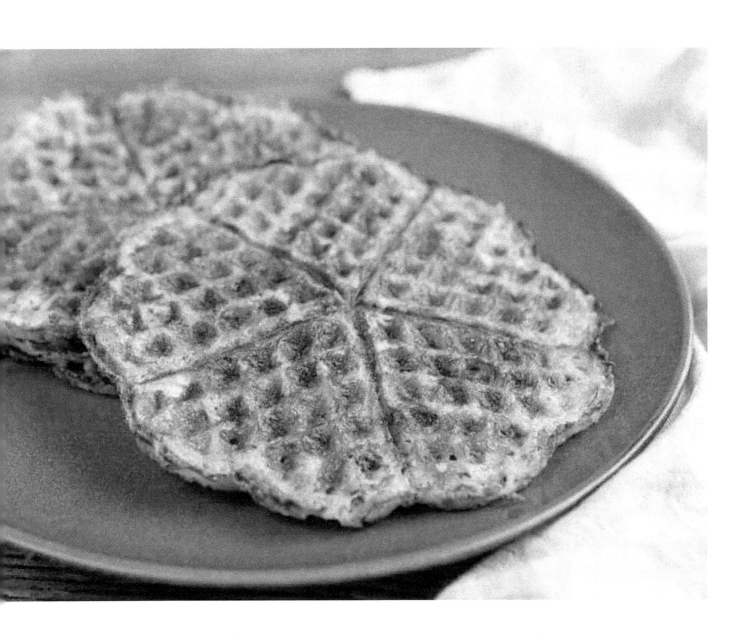

28 Peanut Chaffles

(Ready in about 6 minutes | Serving 2 | Difficulty: Easy)

Per serving: Kcal 264, Fat: 21.6g, Net Carbs: 7.25g, Protein: 9.45g

Ingredients

Chaffle

- 1 Egg
- 1/4 tsp of Baking Powder
- 1 tbsp of Unsweetened Cocoa
- 1 tbsp of Heavy Cream
- 1 tbsp of Powdered Sweetener
- 1/2 tsp of Vanilla Extract
- 1 tsp of Coconut Flour
- 1/2 tsp of Batter Flavor

Butter Filling

- 2 tsp of Powdered Sweetener
- 3 tbsp of Peanut Butter
- 2 tbsp of Heavy Cream

InstructionsPreheat the maker. Combine ingredients of chaffle in a bowl and pour half amount of mixture in maker. Cook for around 5 minutes. Repeat with the rest of the mixture. Blend butter ingredients and spread over chaffles.

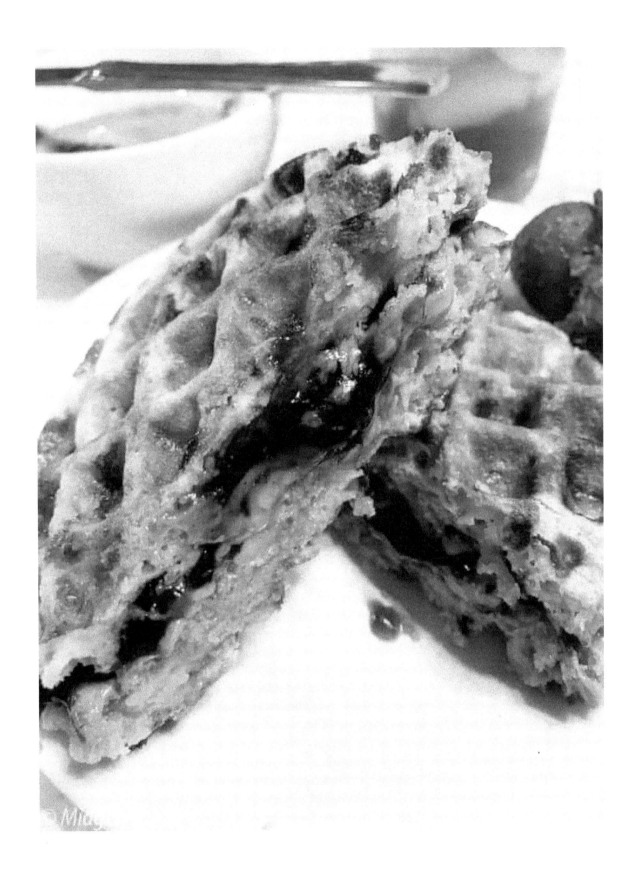

29 Easy Chaffle Recipe

(Ready in about 10 minutes | Serving 2| Difficulty: Easy)

Ingredients
Simple Chaffles

Per serving: Kcal 152, Fat: 8g, Net Carbs: 1g, Protein: 9g

- 1 Egg
- 1/2 Cup of Shredded Cheese Mozarella

Instructions

Add all ingredients to a bowl and whisk to combine. Coat waffle maker using cookir spray and pour half amount of batter into the maker. Cook for around 5 minutes ar repeat with the rest of the batter.

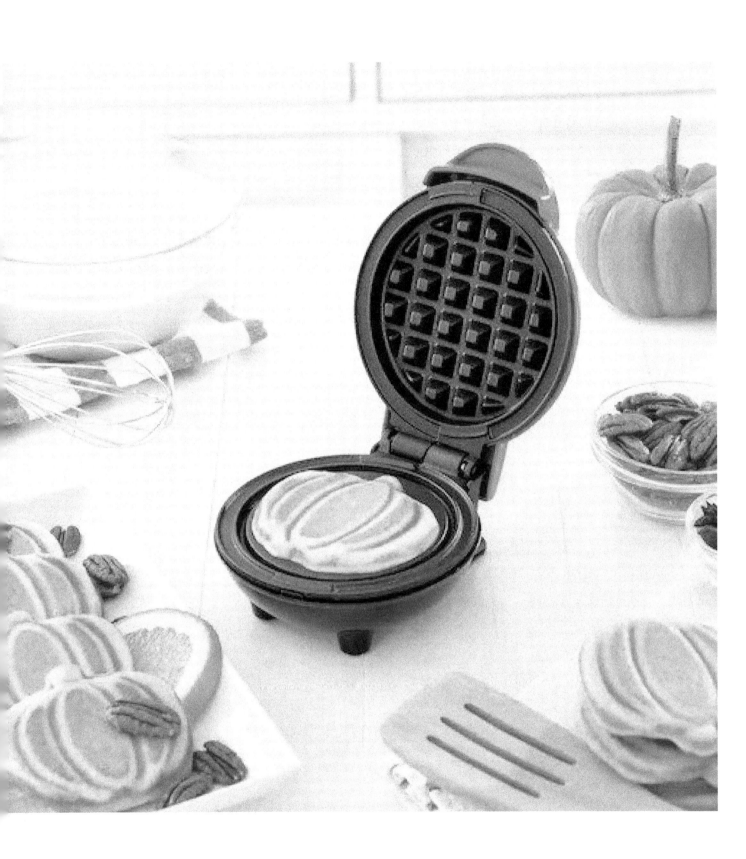

30 Savory Chaffles

Per serving: Kcal 215, Fat: 16.5g, Net Carbs: 2g, Protein: 12g

- 1 Egg
- 1/2 Cup Shredded Cheese Mozarella
- 1/16 Tsp of Xanthan Gum
- 1/4 Cup of Almond Flour

Instructions

Add all ingredients to a bowl and whisk to combine. Coat waffle maker using cooki
spray and pour half amount of batter into the maker. Cook for around 5 minutes a
repeat with the rest of the batter.

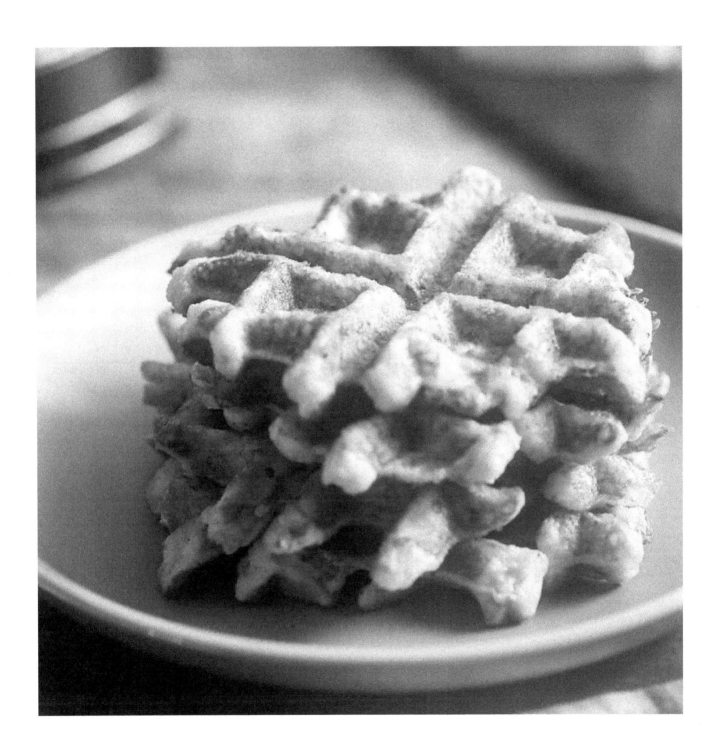

31 Sweet Chaffles

Per serving: Kcal 192, Fat: 15gg, Net Carbs: 1.55g, Protein: 15g

- 1 Egg
- 1/2 Cup of Shredded Cheese Mozzarella
- 1/4 Cup of Almond Flour
- 1/16 Tsp of Xanthan Gum
- 2 Tbsp of Confectioners Swerve

Instructions

Add all ingredients to a bowl and whisk to combine. Coat waffle maker using cookir spray and pour half amount of batter into the maker. Cook for around 5 minutes ar repeat with the rest of the batter.

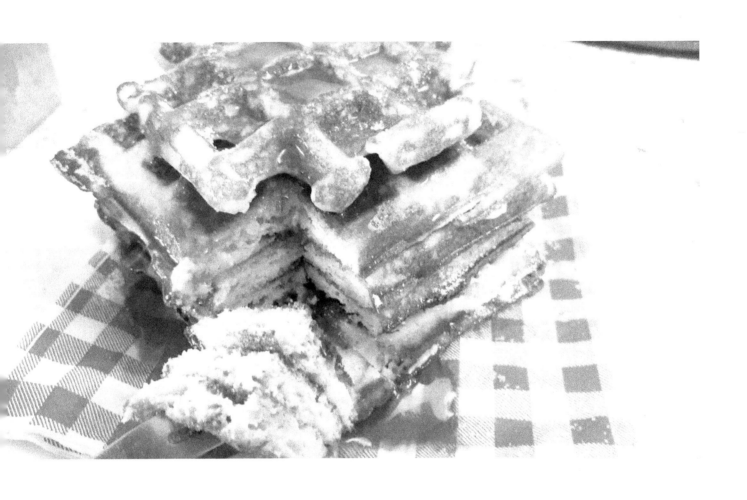

32 Tasty Chaffles

(Ready in about 13 minutes | Serving 2 | Difficulty: Easy)

Per serving: Kcal 116, Fat: 9.5gg, Net Carbs: 2.6g, Protein: 4.5g

Ingredients

- 1 oz softened cream cheese
- 1 tbsp of almond flour
- 1 tbsp of pumpkin puree
- 1 egg
- 1/2 tsp of pumpkin spice

Instructions

Whisk the cream cheese in a bowl. Whisk pumpkin puree and egg in a bowl. A
almond flour and pumpkin spice and mix. Preheat the iron and spray using oil. Po
half amount of mixture in the maker and cook for around 5 minutes. Repeat with t
rest of the batter.

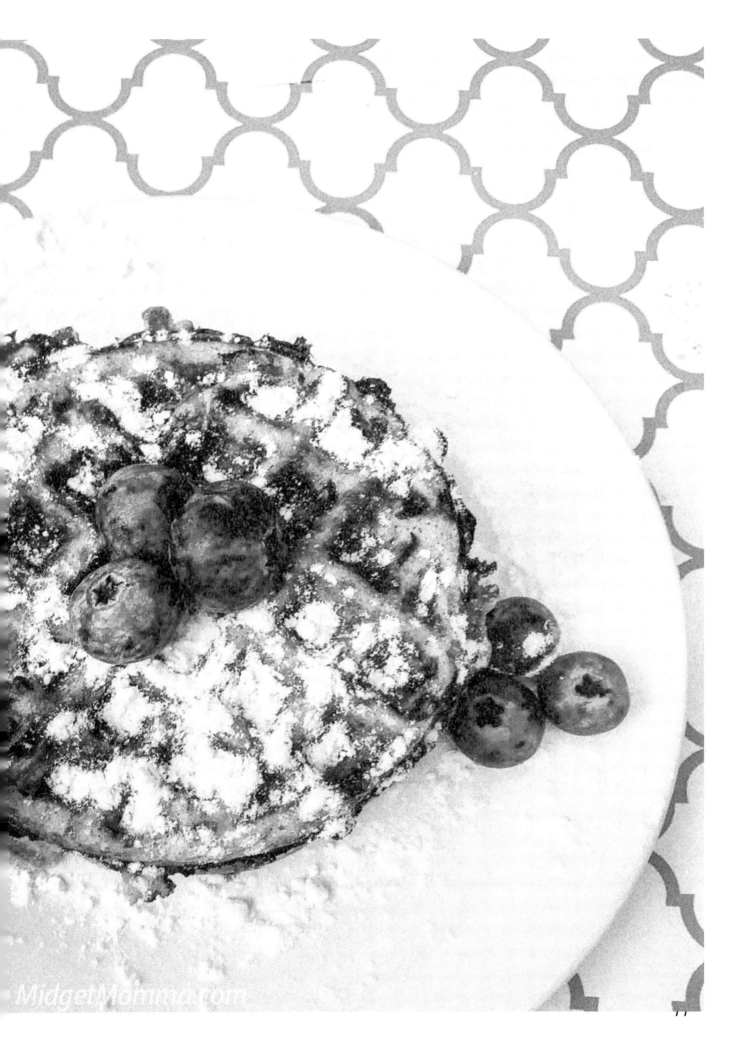

33 Bread Sticks Chaffle

(Ready in about 12 minutes | Serving 7 | Difficulty: Easy)

Per serving: Kcal 80, Fat: 7g, Net Carbs: 1g, Protein: 5g

Ingredients

- 1 egg
- 2 tbsp of almond flour
- 1/2 cup grated mozzarella cheese
- 1/2tsp of garlic powder
- 1/2tsp of salt
- 1/2tsp of oregano

Topping

- 1/2tsp of garlic powder
- 2 tbsp softened butter
- 1/4 cup grated mozzarella cheese

Instructions

Preheat the maker and oil it. Mix all ingredients except topping ingredients. Pour the maker and cook for around 5 minutes. Make four strips of waffle. Mix butter ar garlic powder and coat strips with it. Sprinkle with mozzarella and cook for around minutes.

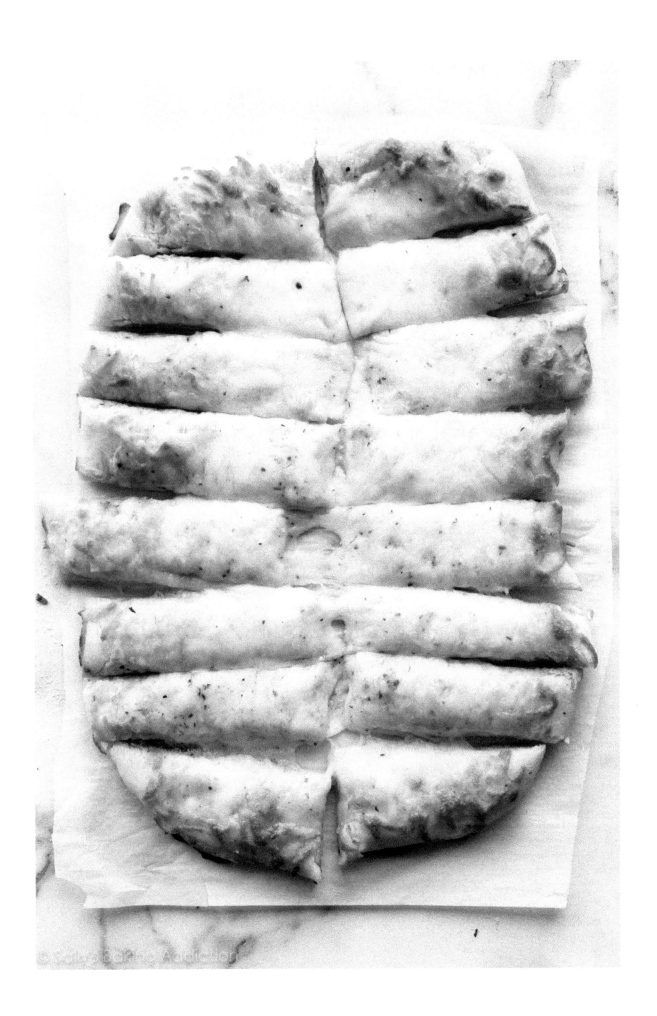

34 Original Chaffle

(Ready in about 5 minutes | Serving 1 | Difficulty: Easy)

Per serving: Kcal 246, Fat: 18g, Net Carbs: 2g, Protein: 17g

Ingredients

- 2 eggs
- 1/4 cup of almond flour
- 1/2 cup of mozzarella
- 1/2 tsp of baking powder

Instructions

Preheat iron and spray with cooking spray. Mix all the ingredients in a bowl and po
half amount of the mixture into the maker. Cook for around 5 minutes and repe
with the rest of the mixture.

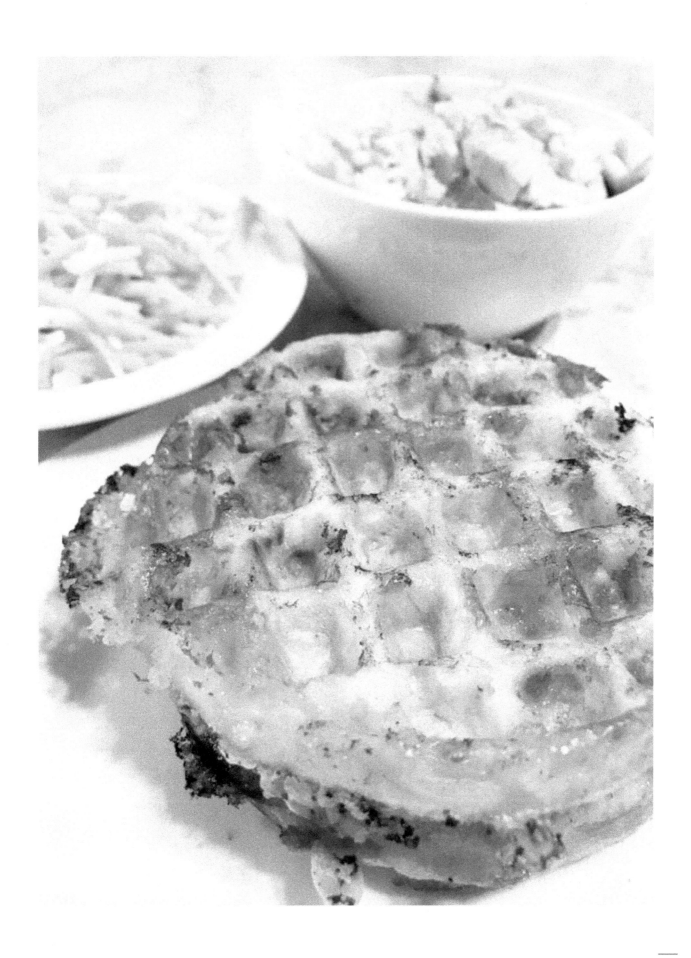

35 Mini Chaffles

(Ready in about 11 minutes | Serving 2 | Difficulty: Easy)

Per serving: Kcal 73, Fat: 6g, Net Carbs: 4g, Protein: 2g

Ingredients

- 2 tsp of Coconut Flour
- 1/4 tsp of Baking Powder
- 4 tsp of Swerve
- 1 Egg
- 1/2 tsp of Vanilla Extract
- 1 oz of Cream Cheese

Instructions

Preheat the iron. Add baking powder, coconut flour and swerve in a bowl and mi

Add cream cheese, egg and vanilla extract in bowl and mix. Pour mixture in the make

and cook for around 4 minutes.

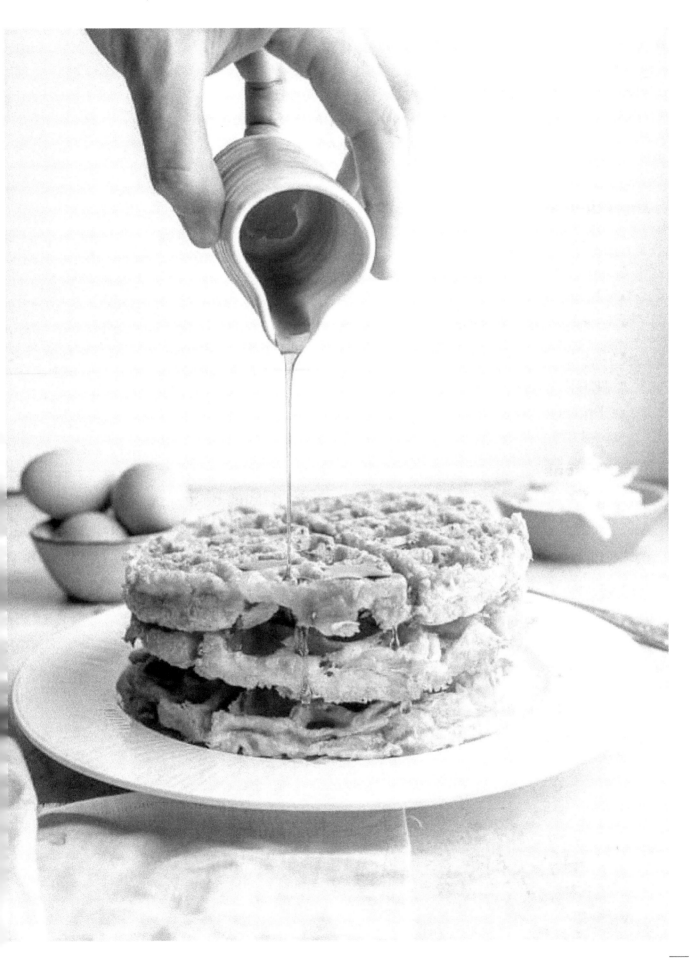

36 Grain-free chaffles

(Ready in about 20 minutes | Serving 2 | Difficulty: Easy)

Per serving: Kcal 277, Fat: 20g, Net Carbs: 4.6g, Protein: 4.8g

Ingredients

- 1 tbsp of almond flour
- 1 tsp of vanilla
- 1 egg
- 1 shake of cinnamon
- 1 cup of mozzarella cheese
- 1 tsp of baking powder
- Butter

Instructions

Mix vanilla extract and egg in a bowl. Mix almond flour, baking powder and cinnamo
Add mozzarella cheese at the end and coat with the mixture evenly. Spray waf
using oil and turn it on. Pour mixture and cook for around 5 minutes. Top with butt
and enjoy.

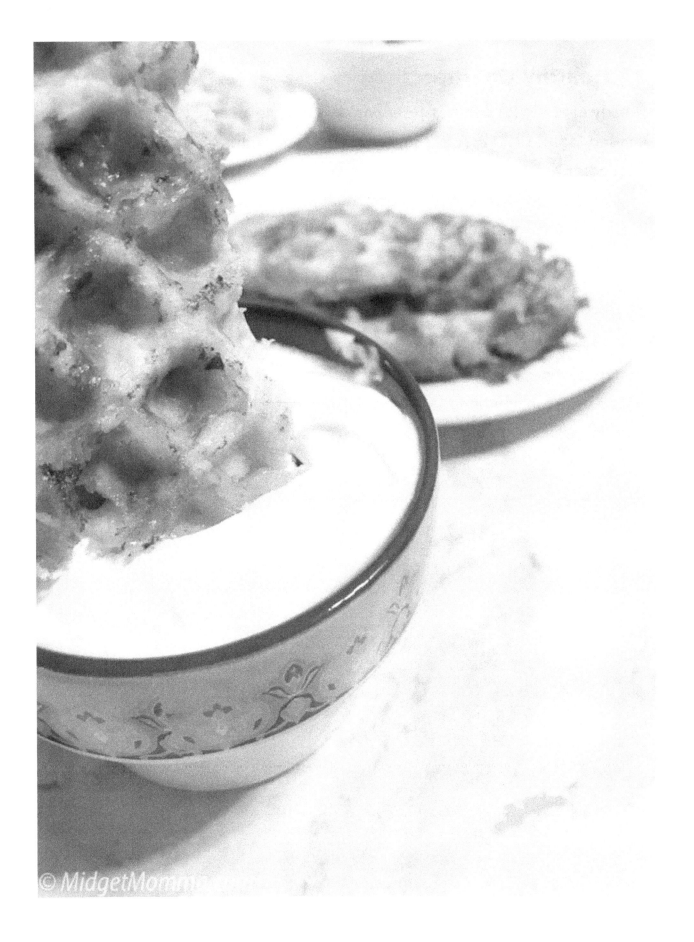

37 Healthy Chaffles

(Ready in about 20 minutes | Serving 4 | Difficulty: Easy)

Per serving: Kcal 411, Fat: 35g, Net Carbs: 6g, Protein: 21g

Ingredients

- 1 1/2 cup of shredded cheese cheddar
- 4 oz. cream cheese
- 4 eggs
- 2 tsp of baking powder
- 1/2 cup of almond flour
- Syrup

Instructions

Oil the waffle maker and mix all ingredients in a bowl. Pour batter into the maker and cook for around 5 minutes. Top with syrup(sugar-free) and enjoy.

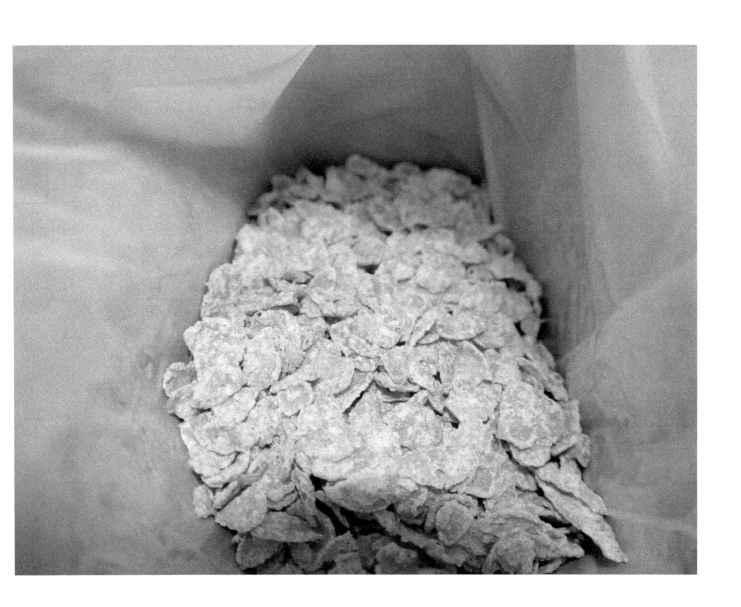

38 Sunny Chaffle

(Ready in about 10 minutes | Serving 1 | Difficulty: Easy)

Per serving: Kcal 320, Fat: 24.3g, Net Carbs: 3.1g, Protein: 21.7g

Ingredients

- 1 egg
- Strawberries
- 2 tbsp of almond flour
- 1/2 cup of mozzarella cheese
- 1/2tsp of baking powder

Instructions

Preheat the maker and mix all the ingredients in a bowl. Pour into the center of the maker and cook for around 5 minutes. Top with strawberries and enjoy.

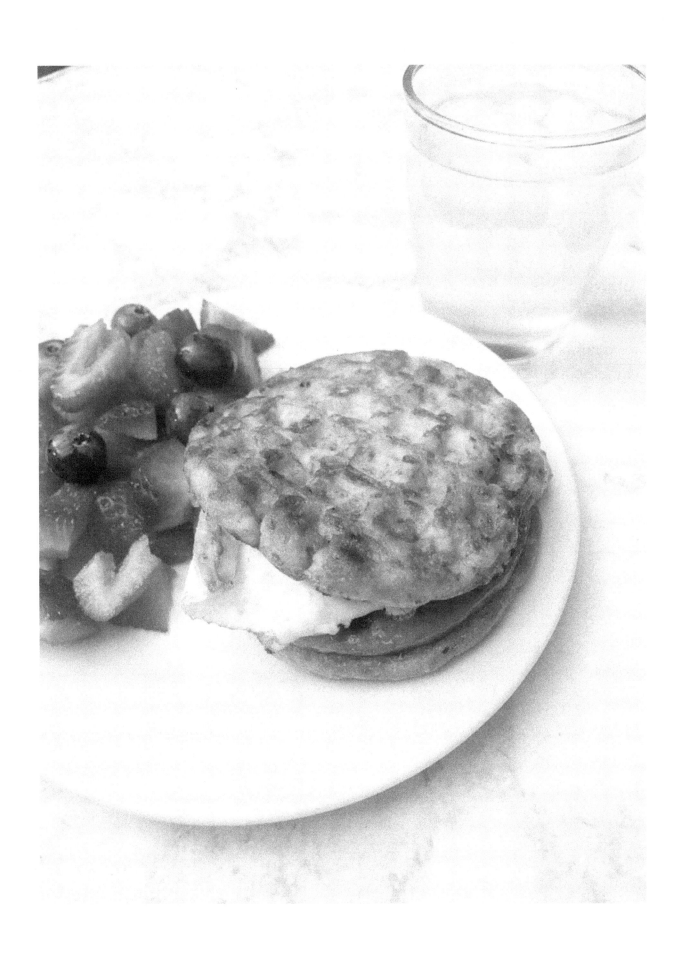

39 Traditional Chaffles

(Ready in about 13 minutes | Serving 1 | Difficulty: Easy)

Per serving: Kcal 291, Fat: 23g, Net Carbs: 1g, Protein: 20g

Ingredients

- 1/2 cup of shredded cheese cheddar
- 1 egg

Instructions

Preheat the maker and oil it gently. Break the egg in a bowl and add the half cup cheddar cheese. Mix and pour half amount of mixture in maker. Cook for around minutes. Repeat with the rest of the mixture.

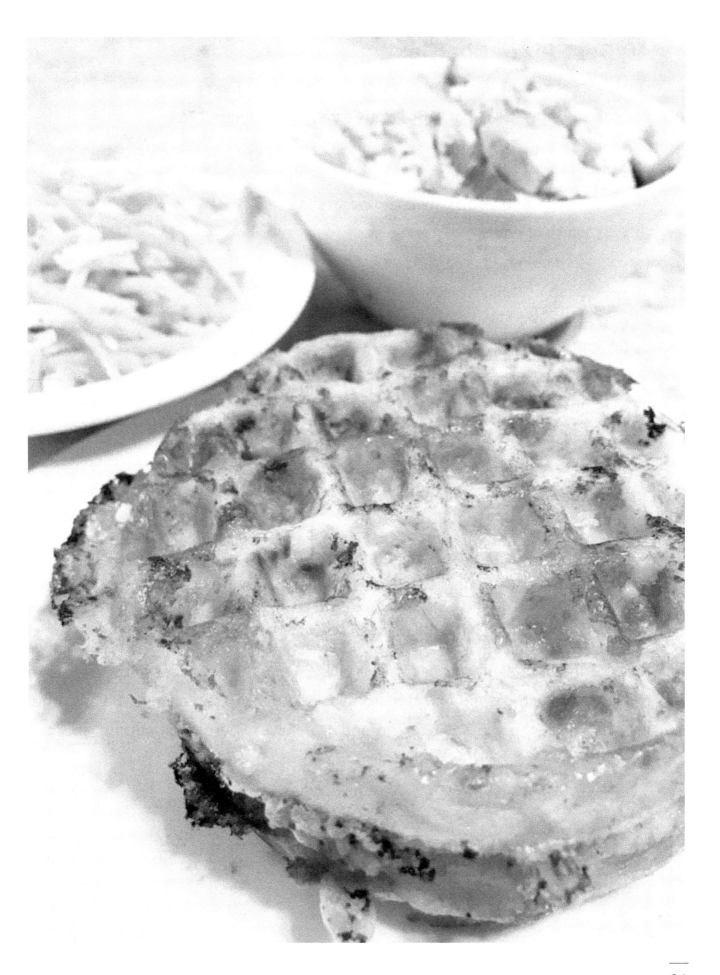

40 Best Pizza Chaffle

(Ready in about 20 minutes | Serving 2 | Difficulty: Easy)

Per serving: Kcal 241, Fat: 18g, Net Carbs: 4g, Protein: 17g

Ingredients

- 1 tsp of coconut flour
- 1/2 cup of shredded cheese mozzarella
- 1 white of egg
- `1 tsp softened cream cheese
- 1/8 tsp of Italian seasoning
- 1/4 tsp of baking powder
- 1/8 tsp of garlic powder
- 3 tsp of marinara sauce
- Salt
- 1/2 cup of mozzarella cheese
- 1 tbsp shredded cheese parmesan
- 6 pepperonis diced in half
- 1/4 tsp of basil seasoning

Instructions

Preheat the oven to 400 degrees F. Preheat the maker as well. Add all the ingredient except pepperoni and parmesan cheese in a bowl and mix. Pour half amount mixture in the maker and cook for around 4 minutes. Repeat with the rest of th mixture. Top with pepperoni, tomato sauce and parmesan cheese. Bake in the ove by placing on the top shelf for around 6 minutes. Turn broil setting and cook f around 2 minutes. Sprinkle with basil.

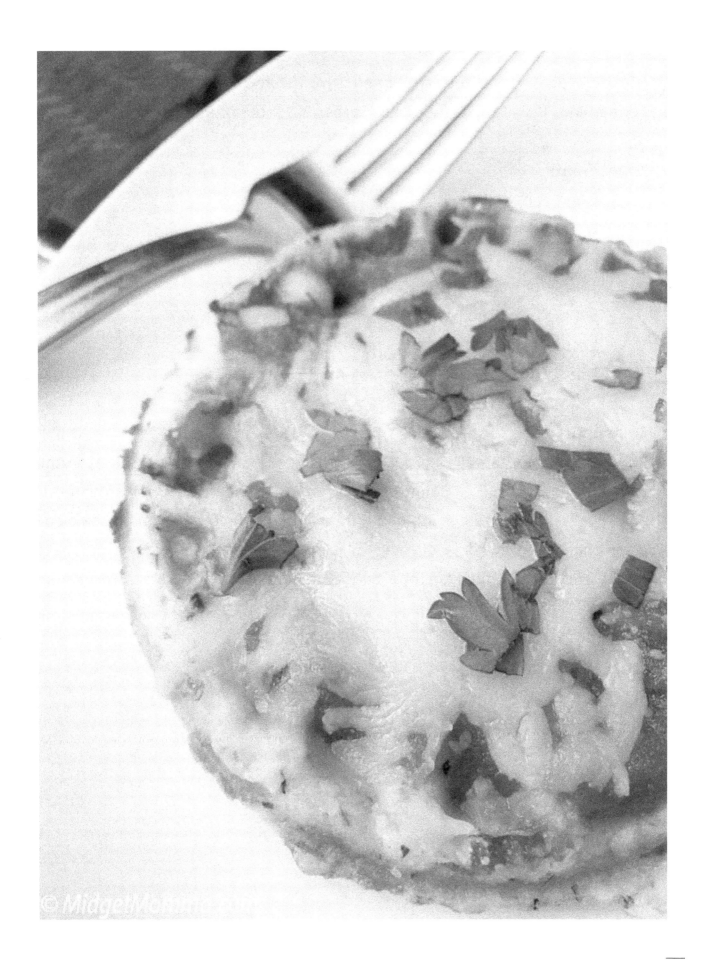

41 Open-Faced Chaffle

(Ready in about 17 minutes | Serving 2 | Difficulty: Easy)

Per serving: Kcal 118, Fat: 8g, Net Carbs: 2g, Protein: 9g

Ingredients

- 1 egg only white
- 1/4 cup shredded cheddar cheese
- 1/4 cup shredded cheese mozzarella
- 3/4 tsp of water
- 1/4 tsp of baking powder
- 1 tsp of coconut flour
- Salt

Instructions

Preheat the oven to 425 degrees F. Preheat the maker as well. Mix everything in bowl and pour half the amount of mixture into a maker. Cook for around 4 minute and repeat with the remaining mixture. Line parchment paper on a cookie sheet ar place chaffles on it. Add a quarter cup of roasted keto beef gravy. Add cheese slic on top and bake in the oven for around 5 minutes in the top rack. Broil for around minute.

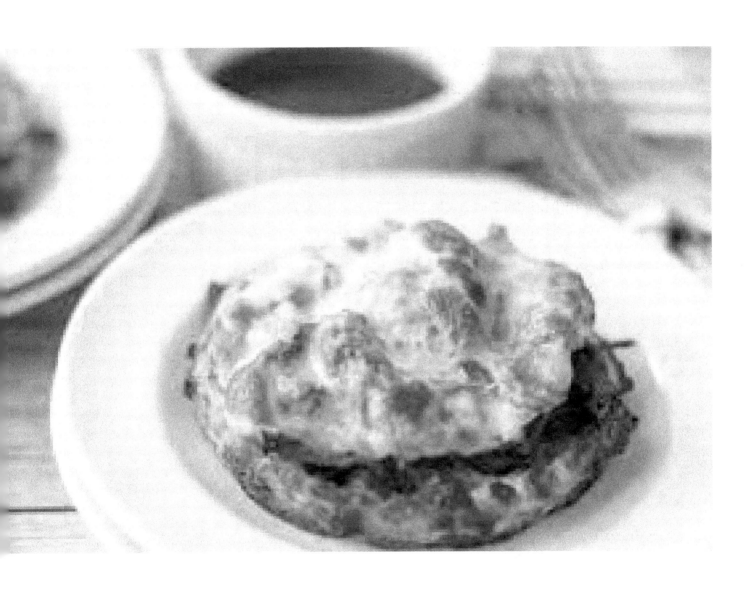

42 Cream Chaffles

(Ready in about 15 minutes | Serving 2 | Difficulty: Easy)

Per serving: Kcal 293, Fat: 27g, Net Carbs: 5g, Protein: 10g

Ingredients

- 4 eggs
- 1 tsp of vanilla extract
- 2 tbsp of melted butter
- 4 oz of cream cheese
- 1 tsp of baking powder

Instructions

Blend all ingredients in a blender for around 1 minute. Spray the waffle maker using cooking spray and pour the mixture into the maker. Cook until it turns crispy and golden.

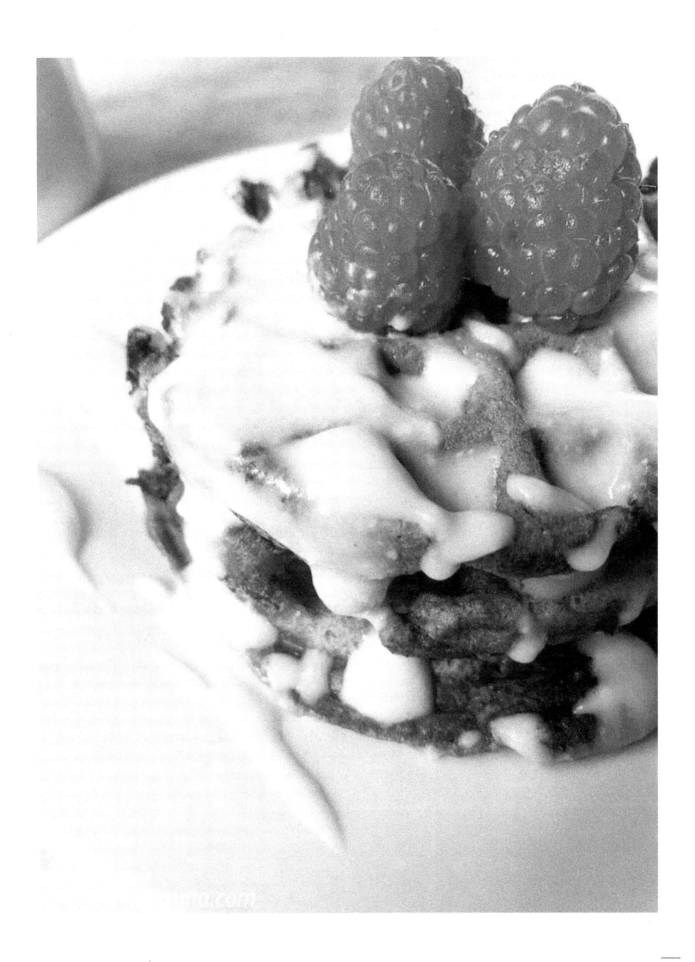

43 Fluffy Chaffles

(Ready in about 45 minutes | Serving 8 | Difficulty: Moderate)

Per serving: Kcal 140, Fat: 11g, Net Carbs: 4g, Protein: 4g

Ingredients

- 64 g of almond flour
- 1 1/2 tsp of baking powder
- 1 tbsp of ground psyllium husk
- 28 g of coconut flour
- 1 tsp of xanthan gum
- 57 g of butter
- 240 ml of water
- 3 tbsp of erythritol
- 3 eggs beaten
- 1/4 tsp of kosher salt
- 1 tsp of vanilla extract

Instructions

Mix flours, xantham gum and husk in a bowl. Warm water, sweetener, salt and butter in a pot and once it starts simmering, add flours and incorporate. Cook for around minutes. Transfer dough to bowl and add egg one by one, mixing using an electric mixer. Add baking powder and vanilla extract and mix. Heat the maker and oil it. Pour batter and cook for around 12 minutes.

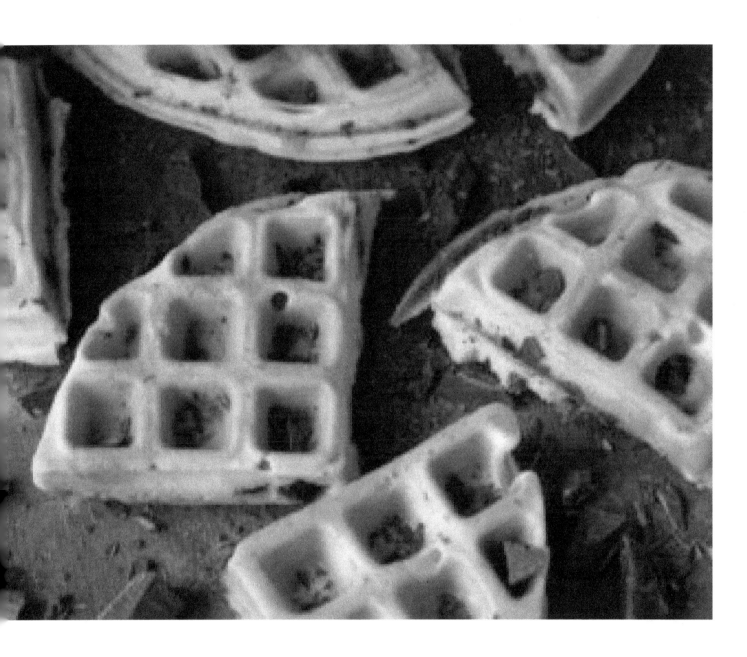

44 Almond Flour Chaffles

(Ready in about 20 minutes | Serving 2 | Difficulty: Easy)

Per serving: Kcal 70, Fat: 3.8g, Net Carbs: 4.9g, Protein: 4g

Ingredients

- 4 separated eggs
- 1/4 cup of granulated Swerve
- 2 cup of almond flour
- 2 tsp of baking powder
- 1/2 cup of butter
- 1 tsp of kosher salt
- 1/2 cup of almond butter
- Cooking spray
- 2 tsp. of vanilla extract
- Maple syrup

Instructions

Preheat waffle maker to high. Mix stevia, almond flour, salt and baking powder in bowl. Melt almond butter and butter in the microwave for around 15 seconds. Stir d ingredients with butter mixture and then add vanilla and yolks. Beat whites in separate bowl and fold in batter. Spray maker using cooking spray and pour t batter. Cook for around 5 minutes. Top with maple syrup and butter.

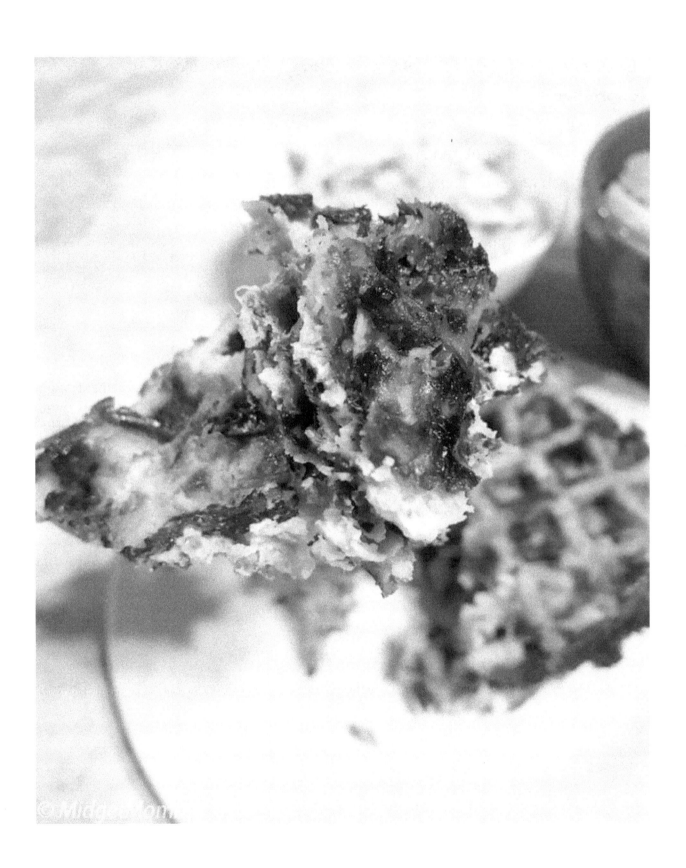

45 Butter Chaffles

(Ready in about 30 minutes | Serving 5 | Difficulty: Easy)

Per serving: Kcal 216, Fat: 19.9g, Net Carbs: 5.5g, Protein: 6.4g

Ingredients

- 5 eggs
- 4 tbsp of granulated sweetener
- 4 tbsp of coconut flour
- 1 tsp of baking powder
- 3 tbsp of milk full fat
- 2 tsp of vanilla
- 125 g of butter melted

Instructions

Beat egg whites in a bowl. Mix yolks with sweetener, baking powder and coconut flour in a separate bowl. Add butter and mix. Add vanilla and milk and mix. Fold whites yolk mixture and pour in maker. Cook for around 5 minutes.

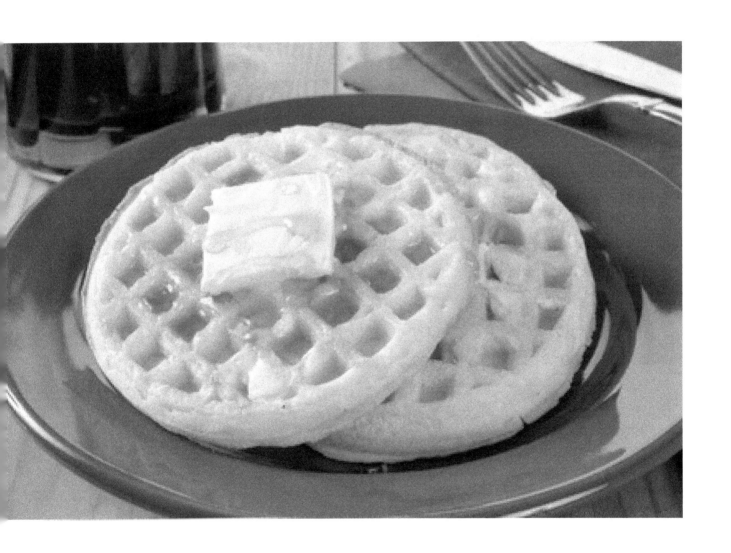

46 Paleo Chaffles

(Ready in about 10minutes | Serving 2 | Difficulty: Easy)

Per serving: Kcal 401, Fat: 37, Net Carbs: 9g, Protein: 13g

Ingredients

- 1 egg
- 2 tbsp of sweetener
- 1/2 cup of Almond Flour
- 1/2 tsp of baking powder Gluten-free
- 2 tbsp of Almond butter
- 1/4 tsp of Sea salt
- 2 tbsp of Butter
- 1/2 tsp of Vanilla extract
- 1/4 cup of almond milk Unsweetened

Instructions

Preheat waffle maker to high temperature. Oil it gently and beat whites in a bow
Combine baking powder, erythritol, salt and almond flour in another bowl. M
almond butter and butter in the microwave and add to the flour mixture. Add yo
vanilla and almond milk and stir. Fold whites in batter and mix. Pour in the mak
and cook for around 5 minutes.

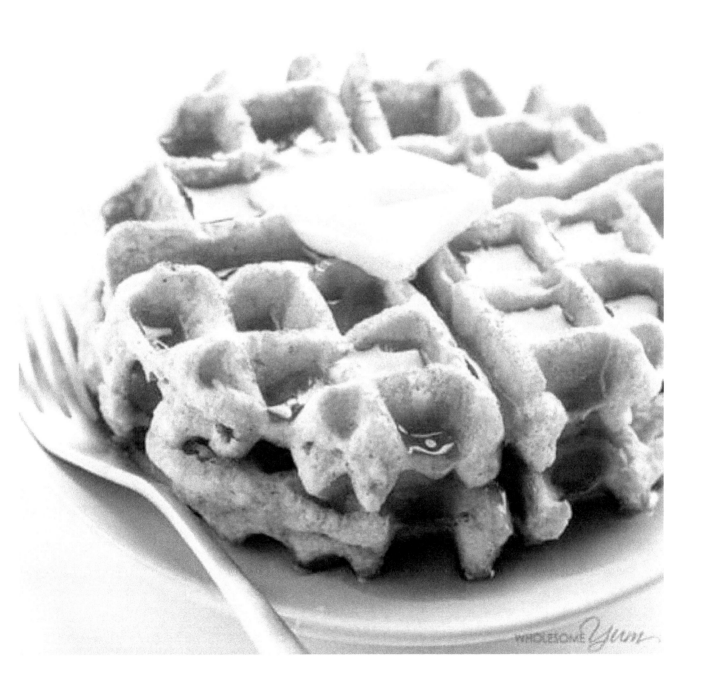

47 Crispy Chaffles

(Ready in about 10 minutes | Serving 4 | Difficulty: Easy)

Per serving: Kcal 64, Fat: 2g, Net Carbs: 4g, Protein: 5g

Ingredients

- 4 tbsp sifted coconut flour
- 1/4 tsp of baking powder
- 1 tsp of coconut oil
- 1 tbsp sweetener granulated
- 2/3 cup of egg whites
- 1/2 tsp of vanilla extract
- 1/4 cup of milk
- 1 tbsp of unsweetened apple sauce

Instructions

Mix sweetener, baking powder and coconut flour in a bowl. Add whites, vanilla, apple sauce and milk in a separate bowl and mix. Pour to the other bowl and form a thick batter. Add oil and spray waffle maker using cooking spray. Once the maker is hot pour the batter and cook for around 4 minutes.

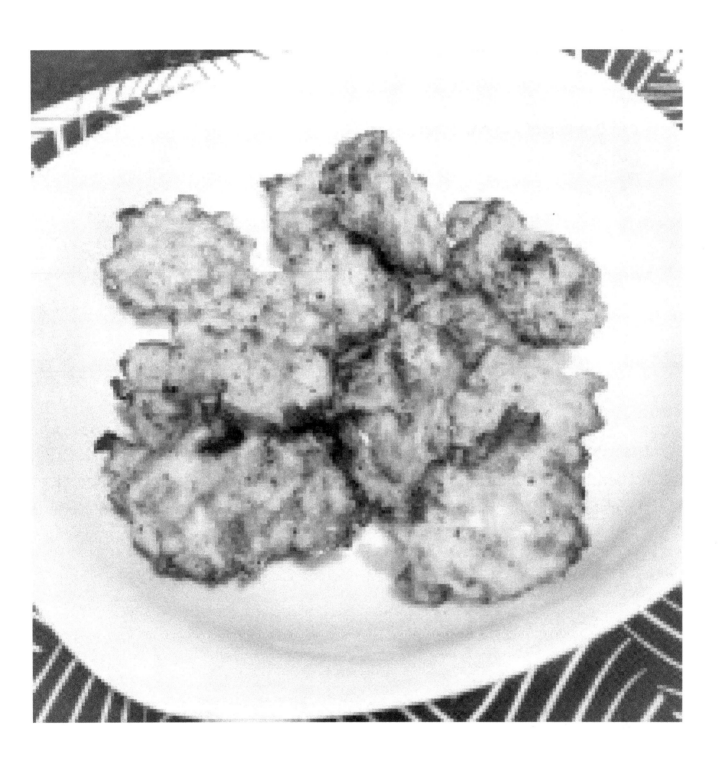

48 Salted Chaffles

(Ready in about 15 minutes | Serving 2 | Difficulty: Easy)

Per serving: Kcal 425, Fat: 36.7g, Net Carbs: 10.7g, Protein: 14.8g

Ingredients

Dry

- 3/4 cup of Almond Flour
- 1 tbsp of Coconut flour
- 2 tbsp of Erythritol
- 1 tsp of Baking Powder
- 1/8 tsp of Himalayan Salt

Wet

- 2 tbsp of Melted Butter
- 2 Eggs
- 2 tbsp of Cream Cheese at room temperature
- 1 tsp of Vanilla Extract

Instructions

Preheat waffle maker to high. Mix wet ingredients in a bowl. Mix dry ingredients in separate bowl. Mix both bowls and pour in the maker. Cook for around 4 minutes.

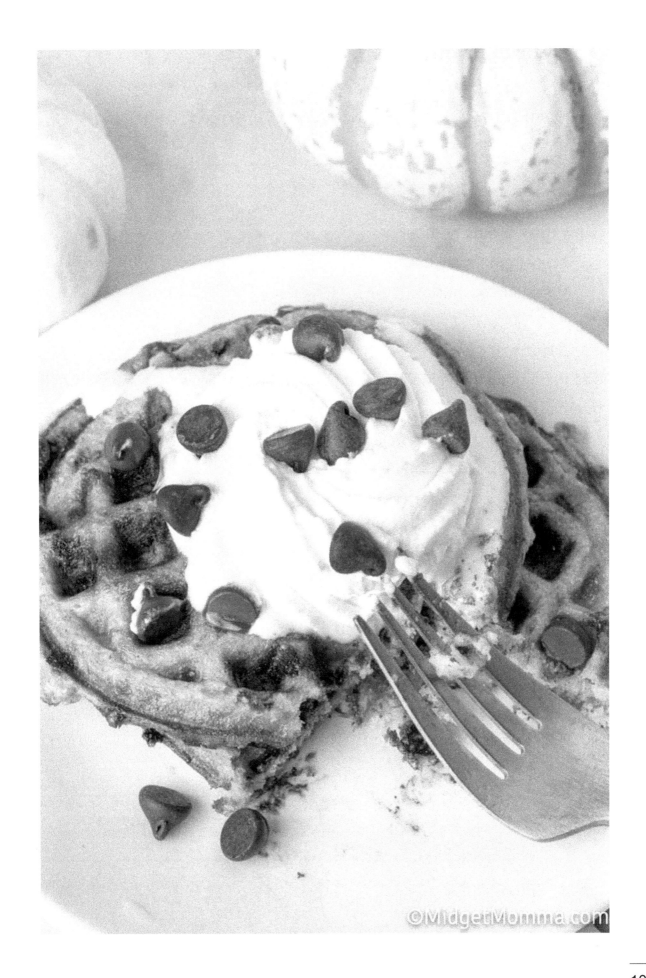

49 Low Carb Chaffles

(Ready in about 8 minutes | Serving 1 | Difficulty: Easy)

Per serving: Kcal 522, Fat: 48g, Net Carbs: 7g, Protein: 19g

Ingredients

- 2 eggs
- 1/2 tsp of baking powder
- 4 tbsp of almond flour
- 2 oz of cream cheese
- 1 tbsp of coconut oil

Instructions

Blend everything in the blender and pour in the maker, which is oiled. Cook for arour 3 minutes.

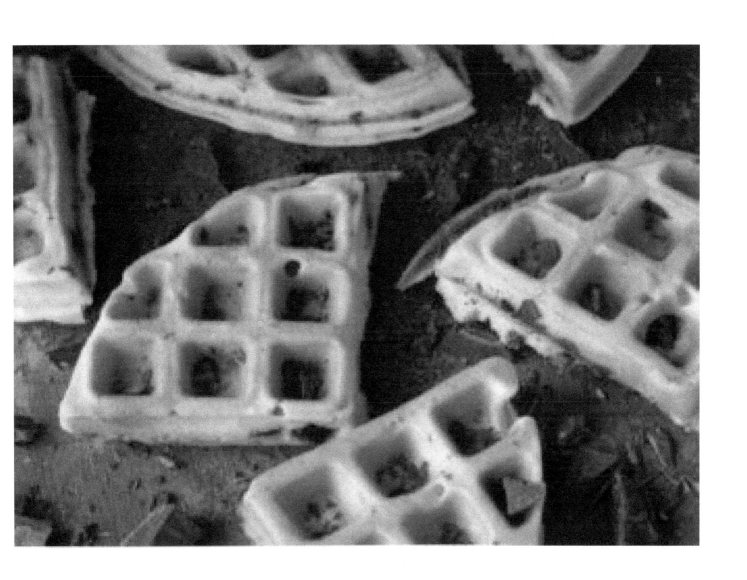

50 Sweet Chaffles

(Ready in about 9 minutes | Serving 2 | Difficulty: Easy)

Per serving: Kcal 331, Fat: 29g, Net Carbs: 7g, Protein: 11g

Ingredients

Dry

- 1/2 cup of almond flour
- 1/2 tsp of sweetener
- 1/4tsp of baking soda
- 1/4tsp of salt
- 1/4 tsp of baking powder
- 1/8 tsp of nutmeg
- 1/4tsp of ground cinnamon
- 1/8 tsp of cloves

Wet

- 2 eggs
- 2 tbsp of melted butter
- 1 tsp of vanilla extract

Instructions

Add dry ingredients to a bowl and mix. Separate yolks and whites in two bowls a[nd] mix butter and vanilla in yolks. Beat whites and add yolks to dry ingredients. Th[en] add whites while mixing gently. Preheat maker to high temperature and pour t[he] mixture. Cook for around 5 minutes.

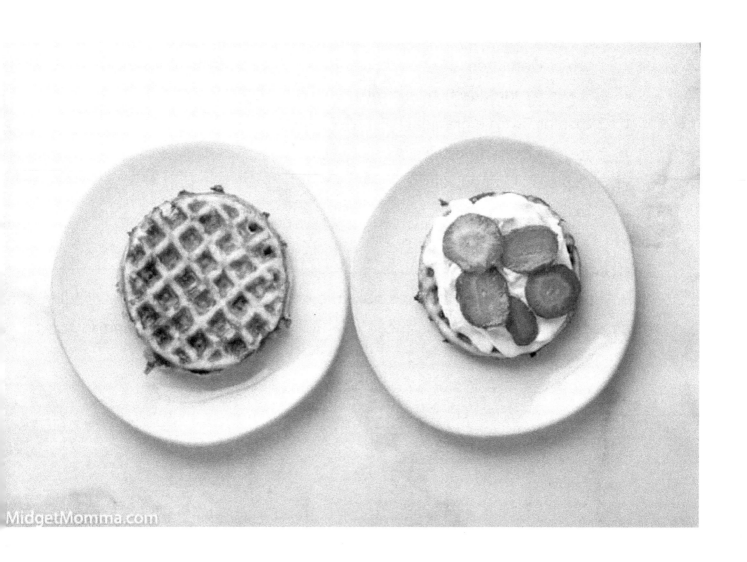

51 Churro Chaffle

(Ready in about 15 minutes | Serving 1 | Difficulty: Easy)

Per serving: Kcal 193, Fat: 14g, Net Carbs: 2g, Protein: 8g

Ingredients

- 1 egg
- 1/4 cup of almond flour
- 1 tsp of cinnamon
- 1/2 cup of shredded cheese mozzarella
- 2 tbsp of Swerve granular
- 2 tbsp of melted butter
- ⅛ tsp of baking powder
- 3 tbsp of Swerve granular

Instructions

Combine everything in a bowl and pour the mixture into the maker by dividing it in
three parts. Melt butter in the meantime in a pan over moderate flame. Add chur
toppings and enjoy.

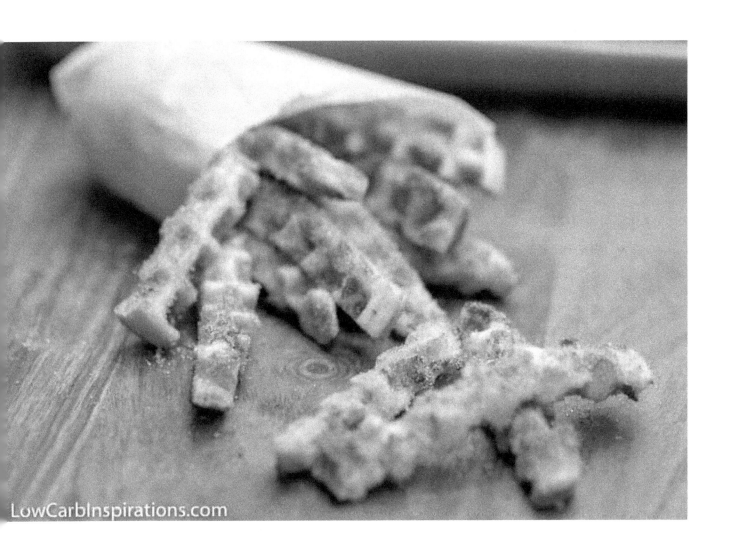

52 Avocado Egg Bake

(Ready in about 20 minutes | Serving 1 | Difficulty: Easy)

Per serving: Kcal 605, Fat: 50.9g, Net Carbs: 18.6g, Protein: 25.3g

Ingredients

- 2 eggs
- 1 avocado, pitted and halved
- ¼ cup of shredded Cheddar cheese
- 1 tbsp. chopped fresh parsley, or according to taste
- Freshly ground black pepper and salt according to taste

Instructions

- Preheat oven to 425 degrees Fahrenheit.
- To make way for one egg, scoop out some of the avocados from where the pit. Put each avocado half on the baking sheet, then crack one egg on to
- Cook for fifteen to twenty minutes in a preheated oven before the egg ready. Season with pepper and salt and finish with Cheddar cheese. Serve with new parsley as a garnish.

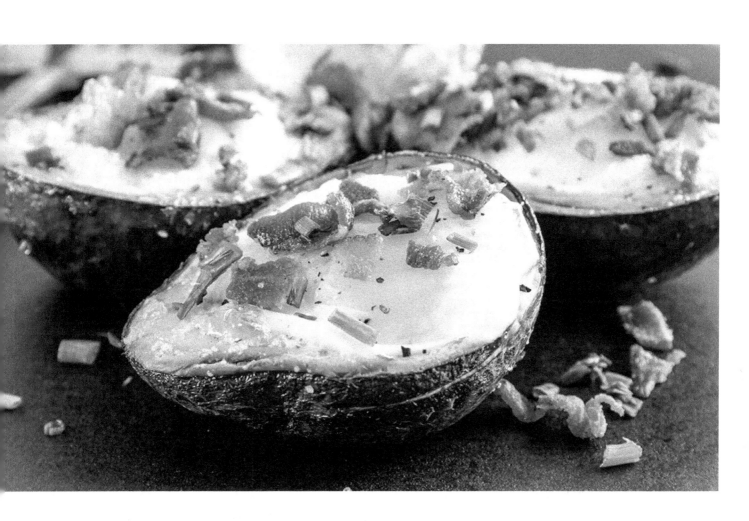

53 Oven-Baked Bacon

(Ready in about 35 minutes | Serving 6 | Difficulty: Easy)
Per serving: Kcal 134, Fat: 10.4g, Net Carbs: 0.4g, Protein: 9.2g

Ingredients

1 (16 oz.) package bacon

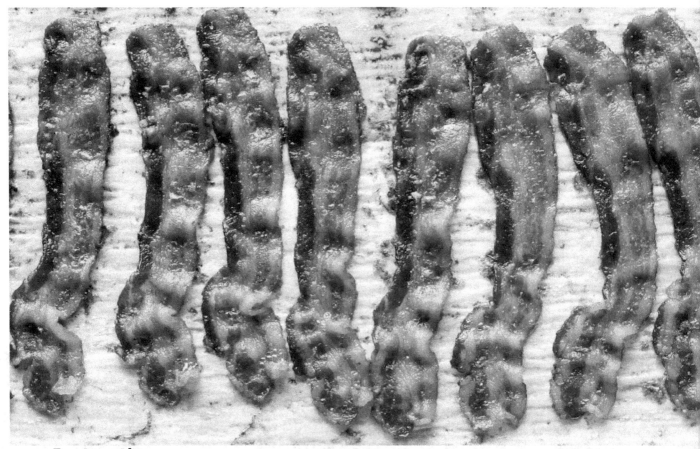

Instructions

- Preheat oven to 350°F. Using parchment paper, line a baking dish.
- Put the bacon slices on a prepared baking sheet, one on top of the other
- Bake for fifteen to twenty minutes in a preheated oven. Take off the dis from the oven. Return the bacon slices to the oven after tossing them wit kitchen tongs. Bake for another fifteen to twenty minutes, or till crisp Thinner slices may require less time to cook, about twenty minutes overa Drain on a paper towel-lined pan.

54 Roasted Leeks With Eggs

(Ready in about 40 minutes | Serving 2 | Difficulty: Easy)

Per serving: Kcal 1219, Fat: 124.6g, Net Carbs: 27.8g, Protein: 11.8g

Ingredients

- 3 green onions
- 2 leeks
- 2 tbsp. melted ghee (clarified butter)
- ¼ tsp. ground black pepper
- ½ tsp. sea salt

Avocado Vinaigrette:

- ¾ cup of light olive oil
- ⅛ tsp. red pepper flakes
- 1 ripe avocado, flesh scooped from the skin, pitted
- 1 lemon, juiced
- Ground black pepper and salt according to taste
- ¼ cup of red wine vinegar
- 1 tsp. olive oil
- ¼ cup of sliced, toasted almonds
- 2 eggs

Instructions

- Preheat oven to 400 degrees Fahrenheit.
- Green tops and bottom half-inch of the leeks should be discarded. Leeks can be sliced in half lengthwise.
- On a sheet tray, arrange the green onions and leeks. Drizzle ghee on top. Season with salt and pepper.
- For fifteen to twenty minutes in a preheated oven, roast till brown.
- In a food processor, thoroughly 3/4 cup olive oil, mix avocado, vinegar, lemon juice, pepper, and salt to make the vinaigrette

- In a skillet on medium-low flame, heat 1 tsp. oil for two to three minute or before whites are just set and the yolks are already runny, break egg onto the opposite sides of the skillet.
- Remove the leeks and onions from the oven and put them on top with tr sunny-side-up eggs. On top, sprinkle red pepper flakes and almonds. Finis with an avocado vinaigrette drizzle.

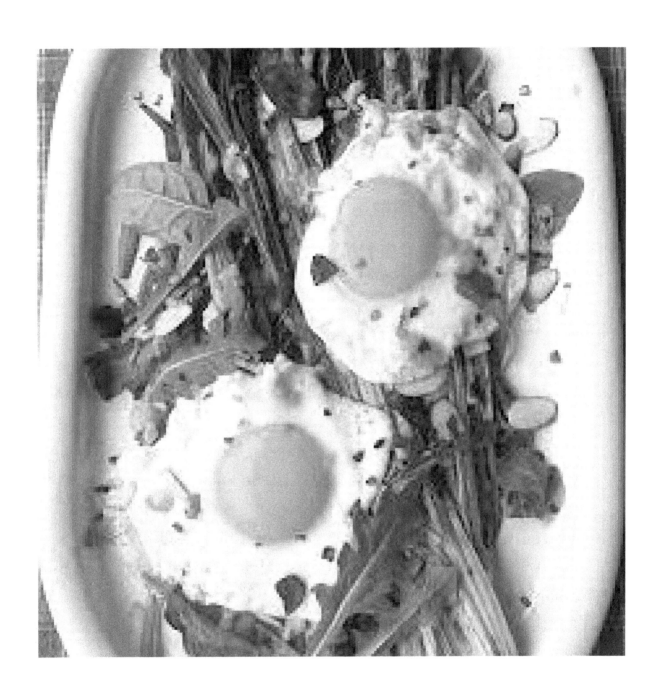

55 Gluten-Free Bagels

(Ready in about 30 minutes | Serving 6 | Difficulty: Easy)

Per serving: Kcal 364, Fat: 27.9g, Net Carbs: 9.7g, Protein: 20.9g

Ingredients

- 1 tbsp. baking powder, gluten-free
- 1 ½ cups of almond flour
- 2 eggs
- 1 tsp. garlic salt
- 2 oz. cream cheese, cubed
- 2 ½ cups of shredded mozzarella cheese

Instructions

- Preheat oven to 400 degrees Fahrenheit. Using parchment paper, line th
  baking sheet.
- In a mixing bowl, add the baking powder, garlic salt, and almond flour.
- In the microwave-safe bowl, mix mozzarella and cream cheese. Microwav
  for one minute, then remove and mix. Microwave for another minute, the
  take it off and stir until all is well combined. Working fast, stir the egg
  and flour mixture into melted cheese mixture. Knead the dough by han
  until it becomes a sticky dough. Continue kneading and pressing the doug
  for approximately two minutes or until it is fully uniform.
- The dough can be divided into six equal bits. Roll each one into the lon
  log, then push the ends together to form a bagel shape and put it on th
  baking sheet that has been prepared.
- For ten to fourteen minutes in the preheated oven, bake till the bagels ar
  golden.

55 Keto Zucchini Hash

(Ready in about 30 minutes | Serving 4 | Difficulty: Easy)

Per serving: Kcal 200, Fat: 17.9g, Net Carbs: 5g, Protein: g

Ingredients

- 3 tbsp. coconut oil
- 4 small zucchini, squeezed dry and grated
- 1 tbsp. butter
- 1 tsp. chili powder, or according to taste
- ⅓ cup of grated Parmesan cheese
- 1 tsp. sea salt
- 2 eggs, beaten
- 1 tsp. cayenne pepper (Optional)

Directions

- In a small skillet over medium flame, combine the coconut oil, butter, and zucchini. Add the chili powder, Parmesan cheese, cayenne pepper, and salt to a mixing bowl. Stir until the cheese has melted.
- Reduce the heat to a minimum and whisk in the eggs before thoroughly combined. Adjust to medium heat and fry, stirring and tossing sometimes, for almost fifteen minutes, or till the edges of hash are lightly browned.

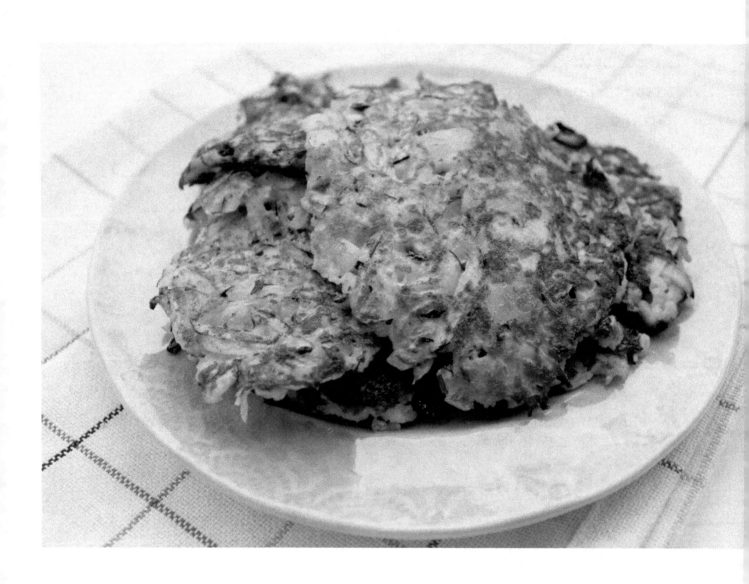

Conclusion

A keto diet may be a healthier option for certain people, although the amount of fat, carbohydrates, and protein prescribed varies from person to person. If you have diabetes, talk to the doctor before starting the diet because it would almost certainly need prescription changes and stronger blood sugar regulation. Are you taking drugs for high blood pressure? Before starting a keto diet again, talk to the doctor. If you're breastfeeding, you shouldn't follow a ketogenic diet. Be mindful that limiting carbs will render you irritable, hungry, and sleepy, among other things. However, this may be a one-time occurrence. Keep in mind that you can eat a balanced diet in order to obtain all of the vitamins and minerals you need. A sufficient amount of fiber is also needed. When the body begins to derive energy from accumulated fat rather than glucose, it is said to be in ketosis. Several trials have shown the powerful weight-loss benefits of a low-carb, or keto, diet. This diet, on the other hand, can be difficult to stick to and can exacerbate health issues in individuals who have certain disorders, such as diabetes type 1. The keto diet is suitable for the majority of citizens. Nonetheless, all major dietary modifications should be discussed with a dietitian or doctor. This is essentially the case with people who have inherent conditions. The keto diet may be an effective therapy for people with drug-resistant epilepsy. Though the diet may be beneficial to people of any age, teenagers, people over 50, and babies can profit the most because they can easily stick to it. Modified keto diets, such as the revised Atkins diet or the low-glycemic index diet, are safer for adolescents and adults. A health care worker should keep a careful eye on someone who is taking a keto diet as a treatment. A doctor and dietitian will maintain track of a person's progress, administer drugs, and test for side effects. The body absorbs fat and protein differently than it does carbohydrates. Carbohydrates have a high insulin reaction. The protein sensitivity to insulin is mild, and the quick insulin response is negligible. Insulin is a fat-producing and fat-conserving enzyme. If you wish to lose weight, consume as many eggs, chickens, fish, and birds as you want, satiate yourself with the fat, and then eat every vegetable that grows on the ground. Butter and coconut oil can be used instead of processed synthetic seed oils. You may be either a sugar or a fat burner, but not both.

CPSIA information can be obtained
at www.ICGtesting.com
Printed in the USA
LVHW061931270621
691285LV00011B/397